To the thousands of patients,
and their families,
who have entrusted me
with their personal spine care.

And to Kathleen Altizer
who has endured and supported me
through this entire challenging project.

A Patient's Guide

Advanced Technologies to Treat Neck and Back Pain

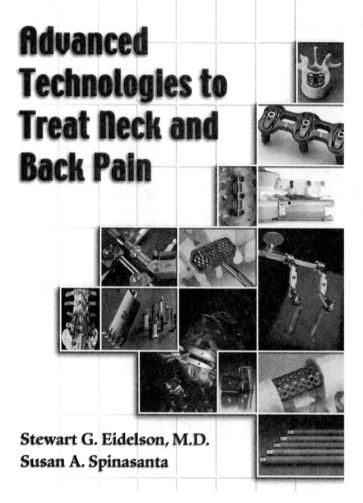

Stewart G. Eidelson, M.D.
Susan A. Spinasanta

Advanced Technologies to Treat Neck and Back Pain, A Patient's Guide

Disclaimer:

Every effort has been made by the authors and contributors to provide the most accurate information possible. Information about products or services contained in this book does not constitute an endorsement of those products or services. This book is not all-inclusive and is not intended to replace the relationship between the reader and their physician, medical professional or other practitioner. The reader assumes all responsibility and risk in the use of the information contained herein. No one associated with the production of this book shall be held responsible for errors, omissions in information herein, or liable for damages resulting in whole or in part from this material.

Publisher:
SYA Press and Research, Inc.
Boca Raton, FL USA
syapress@spineuniverse.com

Copyright© 2005 SYA Press and Research, Inc.
Printed in the United States of America
ISBN <need number>
First printing: March 2005

Library of Congress Cataloging-in-Publication Data
Eidelson, MD, Stewart G.
Spinasanta, Susan A.

Includes biography, illustrations, and index.

Cover design by Larissa Hise Henoch
Inside book design by Dawn Von Strolley Grove

Contents

Contents

Contents

Contents

Contents

Contents

Acknowledgements

This book could not have come to fruition without the dedicated involvement and contributions of many people.

Many of my colleagues contributed to this book and I would like to express my gratitude to everyone and acknowledge Christopher M. Bono, MD; Dana L. Davis, MPT, MTT; Edgar G. Dawson, MD; Richard G. Fessler, MD, PhD; Kevin T. Foley, MD; Steven R. Garfin, MD; Gregory Gilreath, PA-C; Robert E. Isaacs, MD; Laurie Rice-Wyllie, RN, MS, ANPC; Steven H. Richeimer, MD; Gerald E. Rodts Jr., MD; Susan A. Spinasanta; Mary Claire Walsh; Jeffrey C. Wang, MD; Cathleen Zippay, R.EEG/EPT, REDT, CNIM; and Geraldo Zloczover, MD.

Author Biography

Stewart G. Eidelson, MD is an orthopaedic spine surgeon with offices in Boca Raton and Boynton Beach, Florida. In addition to his practice, Dr. Eidelson is the founder of *SpineUniverse.com*, a highly-respected and award-winning educational website for spine patients and health care professionals. His special interest to educate patients about spinal disorders and treatment is further realized in this book.

After receiving his medical degree from Thomas Jefferson Medical College in Philadelphia, PA, he completed an internship at New York Medical College, Metropolitan Hospital in New York, NY. Dr. Eidelson completed an orthopaedic residency at Bailey Seton Hospital (U.S. Public Health Service) in Staten Island, NY and orthopaedic training at the Geisinger Medical Center in Danville, PA and Alfred I. duPont Institute in Wilmington, DE. Further, he completed a Spine Fellowship under Dr. Arthur Steffee at the Cleveland Spine and Arthritis Center in Cleveland, OH.

Dr. Eidelson is a member of many professional societies including the North American Spine Society, American Academy of Orthopaedic Surgeons, Florida Orthopaedic Society, Southern Orthopaedic Society, and the American College of Forensic Medicine.

Throughout his career, Dr. Eidelson has dedicated years to the research, development, and study of outcomes related to surgical procedures to treat spinal disorders. This interest led him to co-found the Palm Beach Orthopaedic and Spinal Research Foundation. His research findings have been published in peer-reviewed journals and presented at society meetings.

Introduction

Stewart G. Eidelson, MD

The advances in the treatment of spinal disorders may best be described as exceptionally remarkable. As an orthopaedic spine surgeon I'm in the front seat of this relatively new frontier of medicine as a physician and in clinical research. That places me in a position to understand the needs of patients and blend my expertise with new technologies to offer treatments that are safer and that afford patients speedier recoveries with better outcomes.

My patients and colleagues know that throughout my career I have been and continue to be an avid advocate for patient education. My advocacy led to the publication of two previous books for patients and the founding of SpineUniverse.com (*www.spine universe.com*), the largest and most visited website dedicated to spinal issues. That leads me to the purpose of this new book, "Advanced Technologies to Treat Neck and Back Pain, A Patient's Guide."

The purpose of this book is to present basic information about spinal disorders and treatment, including some of the newest technological advances. The first part of the book answers questions most patients have about consulting a spine specialist, diagnostic testing, and anatomy. The chapters that follow provide easy to understand information about specific spinal disorders, non-surgical and surgical treatments, and a chapter dedicated to pain management. More than 20 leading spine technology companies have contributed information, illustrations and pictures to help patients better understand current treatment technologies. Further, the entire book is illustrated with more than 180 pictures and includes a glossary and index.

Introduction

It is my hope that the information contained within the covers of this book will assist patients to become better advocates for their own spine care with well-informed and confidence voices.

1

Spine Specialists

Consulting a Spine Specialist: Appointment Preparation and What to Expect

Stewart G. Eidelson, MD

Introduction

B ack and neck pain is the foremost reason why people seek medical attention. For some people, back pain is a one-time inconvenience, while other patients suffer episodic spine problems throughout their life. Approximately 80% of the population in the United States will at some time be affected by back or neck pain. This figure is expected to climb as the population as a whole ages. Often pain is accompanied by other symptoms that include numbness, tingling, and extremity weakness.

Unfortunately there is no 'magic bullet' to halt aging. However, great strides have been made in medicine and the health sciences to increase longevity and expand quality of life. When back or neck pain strikes—it may be wise to seek the opinion of a physician that specializes in spine care. Most patients find a qualified spine specialist through referral from their primary care physician or other treating practitioner.

Spine Surgeons

Orthopaedic spine surgeons and **neurosurgeons** are physicians who have completed additional years of medical training to diagnose and treat disorders affecting the spine. Often these specialists have received advanced training such as a fellowship in spine care. Spinal disorders include **scoliosis** (sko-lee-oh-sis), **osteoarthritis** (os-t-o-arth-rye-tis), **osteoporosis** (os-t-o-pour-o-sis), **herniated disc** (her-knee-ate-ed disc), **spinal stenosis** (spinal sten-oh-sis), trauma, **vertebral fracture,** deformity, tumor, infection, and congenital abnormalities.

Appointment Preparation

Consulting a spine specialist is similar to a visit with a primary care physician (PCP)—except the focus is on the spine. The consultation includes a physical and neurological examination and review of the patient's medical history and current symptoms. The following suggestions are provided to help patients prepare:

1. Write down your medical history, family history and all medications including over-the-counter drugs, vitamins and herbs. Include allergies and side effects experienced from medications (or other substances) taken in the past.
2. List all symptoms. Describe the type of pain, location, when it started and activities that aggravate or alleviate symptoms.
3. Bring a copy of reported results from diagnostic tests or studies (e.g. x-ray, blood work). If possible, bring the actual x-ray, MRI, CT Scan, or other imaging study/film.
4. List the names and contact information of other medical professionals or practitioners who are currently treating or who have treated the condition.
5. Write down questions and concerns.
6. Bring an extra set of 'ears' such as a family member or friend to the consultation.

What to Expect

New patients complete forms to provide information about their medical and family history, previous surgery/ies, allergies, and current medications. A universal pain diagram is provided to help the patient illustrate the location and characteristics of their pain. The diagram is a drawing of the front and back of the body. The patient indicates where pain is felt using symbols, grades the intensity and type of pain, as well as other sensations such as numbness or weakness.

Prior to meeting the spine specialist, the medical assistant or nurse may weigh the patient, measure height, and take the patient's blood pressure and pulse. The spine specialist will review the written information provided by the patient and ask many questions. Questions may include:

- When did the symptoms begin?
- Was the onset of symptoms gradual or sudden?
- Does the pain radiate into the arms or legs (extremities)?
- Was there a specific event such as a car accident that preceded the symptoms or is this a recurring problem?
- How does the condition affect your life? For example, does it prevent you from working, driving a car, walking, or other daily activities?

Physical Examination

Prior to the examination, the patient changes into a gown. The physician inspects and feels (called '**palpation**', pal-pay-shun) the spine for muscle tenderness and spasm. With the patient standing, the shoulders and hips are checked to determine if they are of equal height bilaterally (left, right sides). Spinal range-of-motion is evaluated as the patient turns their head from side-to-side; bends their head toward the shoulder; twists the shoulders from side-to-side; bends forward at the waist to touch their toes, from side-to-side, and then backward.

3

While the patient is lying on their back (called 'supine', sue-pine), the physician may raise each of the patient's legs—this test is called straight leg raises. Each straight leg raise may be combined while the patient **dorsiflexes** (door-see-flexes) the foot (toes pointed toward the head). Further, each leg is measured to determine if the legs are of equal size and length.

Neurological Examination

The findings from the physical examination determine the extent of the motor and sensory evaluation. Typically, a neurological examination may include:

1. The patient walks back and forth, heel-to-toe, on tip-toe and on the heels. During these exercises, the physician observes the patient's posture, balance, and extremities (arms, legs) during movement.
2. Balance is observed as the patient stands with both feet together without arm support. This test (called the Romberg Test) is repeated with the eyes open and closed.
3. The physician provides resistance against the patient's force. For example, with the patient seated, the patient lifts their left knee and tries to hold it up against the gentle downward force exerted by the physician's hand. Resistance exercises test muscle strength, flexion and extension.
4. A pinwheel instrument is gently moved across the same area of each leg (e.g. calf, thigh) to determine if the patient feels the same sensations in each leg. A tuning fork may be used to determine if the patient perceives vibration.
5. A rubber-tipped reflex hammer is gently tapped against one or more tendons in the arms or legs (e.g. elbow, knee). The reflexes can be tested when the patient is sitting or standing.
6. The physician moves his finger up, down, and from side-to-side to test the patient's ability to follow the movement with their eyes.

Conclusion

Each piece of information obtained from the patient about their condition is used to form the diagnosis and to determine the next step in the patient's care. Sometimes further diagnostic testing is required to confirm the physician's findings or to provide more information about the extent of the patient's spinal disorder.

2

Diagnostic Studies

Diagnostic Tests: A Synopsis

Stewart G. Eidelson, MD

F ortunately, most spinal disorders are more painful than serious! A sprain or strain is an example of a painful condition that is relatively easy to treat. Even in cases where a **sprain** or **strain** is suspected as the cause of discomfort, the treating physician may order a standard x-ray to rule out a more serious disorder such as a fracture.

Of course not all neck and back disorders are easy to diagnose. Some disorders require diagnostic testing to determine the next step—the proper treatment. Listed below in alphabetical order are the more common diagnostic tests used by spine specialists.

A **Bone Density Scan** is also called a **Bone Mineral Density (BMD)** test. The purpose of this test is to measure the compactness of bone. It is often used to help to prevent and diagnose **osteoporosis** (os-t-o-pour-o-sis). Computerized scanning equipment uses a low dose of radiation to measure the density of the hip and lower spine. The test takes about 15 minutes.

A Bone Scan is used to detect fine stress fractures, arthritis, infection and tumors. Prior to the test, the patient is injected with a liquid radioactive tracing element called a **nuclide** (noo-clid). The nuclide is allowed to collect in the bones for two to four hours. Thereafter, the patient lies on the scanning table and a gamma ray scanner moves back and forth over the entire body.

The results of the bone scan reveal hot and cold spots. A hot spot denotes an area of high tracer uptake and a cold spot, less. Sometimes a bone scan can detect certain spinal abnormalities weeks before it could be found on a traditional x-ray.

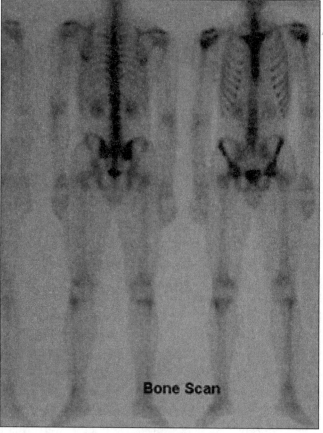

Bone Scan
© SpineUniverse.com. Used with permission.

CT Scan (Computerized Axial Tomography) or **CAT Scan** was developed in 1970. The CT Scan evolved from tomograms; multiple x-rays taken at different levels to determine the depth of an abnormality. With the advent of computers in medicine, study times are shorter with less exposure to radiation.

The CT Scan has become an important adjunct to x-rays. The CT Scan utilizes multiple x-ray beams projected at angles in combination with computer resources to create detailed three-dimensional cross-sectional images. Each image or picture resembles a slice of tissue at a different depth or level.

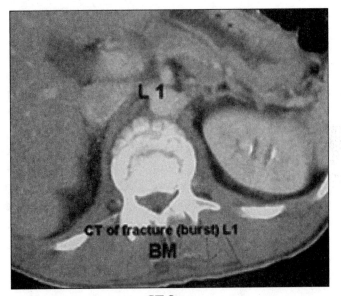

CT Scan
Axial view (overview) of a vertebral fracture.

© SpineUniverse.com. Used with permission.

Electromyography (EMG) (elec-tro-mypah-gra-fee) is a nerve function test performed to determine if muscle function is normal or abnormal. EMG tests the nerve impulse originating from the brain and spinal cord. The nerve pulse is followed enroute to its final destination to determine if the nerve impulse is blocked or delayed and where. Sometimes an EMG is performed with a **Nerve Conduction Velocity (NCV)** test.

Discography (dis-ah-gra-fee) or a **discogram** is a type of x-ray study used to analyze the intervertebral disc space. The abnormal disc is injected with an illuminating contrast fluid under x-ray guidance. As the fluid is injected, pressure increases within the disc that may replicate the patient's symptoms including leg pain. A discogram aids in the detection of spinal abnormalities related to disc function and anatomical disorders.

Laboratory Tests

Blood test results may reveal infection or tumor—disorders that may not be readily found on an x-ray. **Urinalysis** (yu-ri-nal-is-sis) may reveal kidney stones, which may cause severe back pain. Further, urinalysis can detect by-products created when muscle breaks down sometimes due to trauma or disease.

MRI (Magnetic Resonance Imaging) is one of the most sensitive diagnostic tools first used on humans in 1971. MRI is radiation-free; quite different from an x-ray or CT Scan. The MRI equipment is primarily comprised two ultra powerful magnets; one external and one internal.

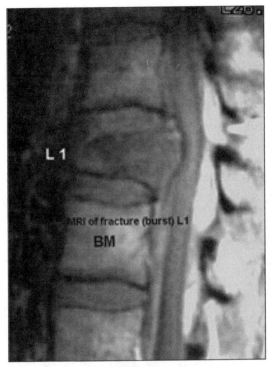

MRI
Lateral (side) view of a vertebral fracture.
© SpineUniverse.com. Used with permission.

The human body contains millions of negative- and positive-charged atoms. When these atoms are exposed to the MRI's electro-magnetic waves, the atoms act like mini-magnets. During the test, a computer collects and combines data that is further manipulated using complex mathematical equations. The final product is a highly detailed film image of the patient's anatomy. MRI is the 'gold standard' in imaging and is best suited for evaluating soft tissue disorders involving the spinal cord, nerves, and intervertebral discs.

To appreciate the difference between an x-ray and an MRI image—consider the finished quality of an imaged intervertebral disc. Under x-ray, an intervertebral disc appears as a pocket of air. In contrast, the MRI image of the same disc includes detail about existing structural deformities or problems such as a disc bulge or rupture (herniation). Additionally, an MRI reflects how the deformity affects the surrounding structures (e.g. nerve impingement). Further, the use of contrast dye administered intravenously to the patient further defines and highlights particular aspects of the spinal anatomy.

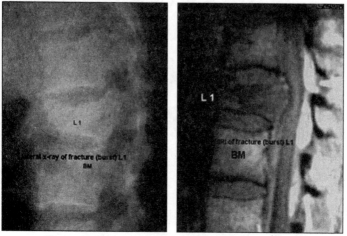

**X-ray (left) versus MRI (right). Images reflect
a lateral (side) view of a vertebral fracture.**

© SpineUniverse.com. Used with permission.

MRI is not perfect science and has drawbacks. Patients with internal ferromagnetic (metallic iron) devices such as a pacemaker, metal cardiac valve or metal in the examination area cannot undergo MRI. The powerful MRI magnets will interfere with metallic devices. In these patients a CT Scan is performed. Newer types of MRI equipment are ideal for **claustrophobic** (claw-stro-foe-bick) patients. The open-air design eliminates the need for confinement within an imaging tube.

Sometimes an MRI creates a false positive. This means the MRI revealed a disorder for which the patient has no symptoms. A bulging disc is an example. There are people who have a bulging disc but are unaware of its existence because they have no pain or other symptoms. In fact, if an MRI was performed on 100 people without neck or back pain, 20-25% may be found to have a disc disorder or arthritic condition. This does not mean that just because an abnormality was detected that treatment is required. The point is that the patient's symptoms must coincide with the test results for an accurate diagnosis.

Nerve Conduction Velocity (NCV) is sometimes performed with an **EMG (Electromyography)** study. NCV stimulates a specific nerve and records the nerve's ability to transmit an impulse. The results of the study may help to reveal where a particular nerve is unable to function normally.

X-Ray or **radiographs** are still the most common test performed today. The x-ray was discovered in 1895 by Wilhelm Conrad Roentgen. His remarkable achievement radically changed the practice of medicine. For the first time physicians could see beneath the skin and underlying soft tissues to the skeleton without autopsy. Roentgen did not entirely understand the unusual rays and therefore used the letter 'x' as a description. In Algebra 'x' refers to an unknown.

When the spine is x-rayed the beams pass through the skin, muscle, tendons and ligaments (soft tissues). Upon meeting bone, the beams stop and create a white shadow on the film. A bony abnormality is reflected on the finished film. Shades of gray mirror the different tissue densities. X-rays are best for viewing bone and are not helpful for finding soft tissue trauma.

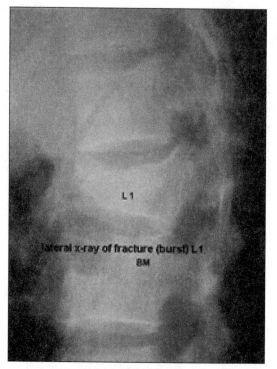

X-Ray (Radiograph)
Lateral (side) image of a vertebral fracture.
© SpineUniverse.com. Used with permission.

X-rays are not performed at random and are ordered when spine or extremity pain (arm, leg) is severe, chronic or progressive. An x-ray may help to rule out particular problems that involve bone and some soft tissue disorders. If an x-ray is not conclusive, additional tests may be ordered, especially if something suspicious is detected on the x-ray.

Conclusion

Diagnostic tests are a valuable tool spine specialists use to prevent, monitor and treat disorders. Although not discussed here, spine surgeons rely on diagnostic tests as a pre-operative planning tool.

Signa OpenSpeed 0.7T: Magnetic Resonance Imaging

GE Healthcare

Magnetic Resonance Imaging (MRI) is a diagnostic imaging technology. The system uses a powerful magnet, radiofrequency waves, and computer to produce detailed pictures of a patient's anatomy. MR is used to image the central nervous system, joints, arms and legs, vascular system—in fact, the entire body!

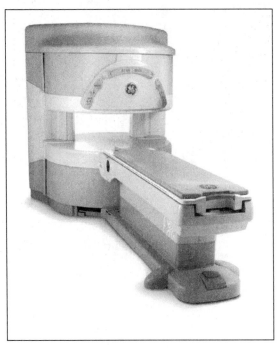

Signa OpenSpeed 0.7T

©GE Healthcare. Used with permission.

GE Healthcare's Signa OpenSpeed system is an open MRI system. It provides a comfortable environment for patients who require MR examination. The Signa OpenSpeed's spacious opening is ideal for patients who are claustrophobic. Unlike MRI of yesterday, the Signa OpenSpeed is "ultra low noise". Other patient-friendly comfort features include adjustable lighting and airflow and ease in summoning assistance.

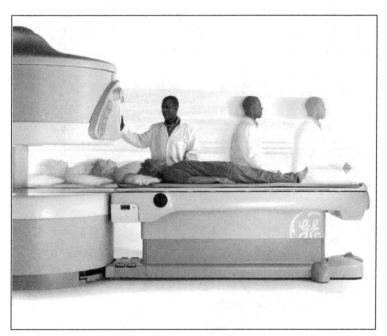

Signa OpenSpeed 0.7T.
The table bed is adjustable.

© GE Healthcare. Used with permission.

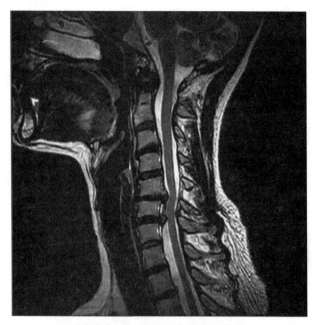

**MRI Study: Lateral (side) view
of a patient's cervical spine.**

© GE Healthcare. Used with permission.

3

Anatomy

Spinal Anatomy: A Synopsis

Stewart G. Eidelson, MD

This chapter is an introduction to the basic components of the spine. The goal is to provide the reader with a foundation of knowledge from which to better understand the material presented in subsequent chapters.

To begin, the spine is part of the body's **musculoskeletal** system, which means muscle and bone. The **skeleton** is the body's framework or scaffolding system. Skeletal bones are classified as long, short, flat or irregular and vary in length, width and depth. The bones in the spine are irregular in shape and provide places to connect to other bones. The purpose of the skeletal system is to support the body against the force of gravity, protect soft tissues, produce red blood cells, store inorganic calcium and phosphorus salts, and to provide sites for muscle attachment to enable body movement.

Bone is a living tissue. During prenatal development bones are **cartilaginous** (car-t-lay-gin-us). A newborn baby's body may contain more than 300 cartilaginous bones that gradually fuse to form approximately 206 permanent bones by adulthood. **Osteoblasts** (os-t-o-blasts) help form bone and **ossification** (os-efik-kay-shun) hardens bone.

The interior bone tissue resembles reinforced concrete. **Collagen** (call-ah-gin) threads made of fibrous protein reinforce the hard cement formed by calcium and phosphorus compounds. Concentric rings of bone fibers called **Haversian spaces** (hav-er-sh-on spaces) surround canals that contain nerve fibers and blood vessels. **Osteocytes** (os-t-o-sites) are cells that help to maintain bone structure. During adulthood, bone continually rejuvenates itself by breaking down and rebuilding. **Osteoclasts** (os-t-o-kasts) break bone down and **osteoblasts** (os-t-o-blasts) return to build new bone. Calcium is very important to the action of the osteoblasts.

The **spinal column** is also called the **vertebral column.** The bones in the spine are called **vertebrae** (ver-ta-bray). **Vertebra** (ver-ta-bra) refers to one spinal segment or level and vertebrae means more than one (ver-ta-bray). The spinal column begins at the base of the skull and continues to the pelvis. Alternate layers of bone (vertebrae) and **cartilage** (car-til-ledge)—the **intervertebral discs**—stack vertically one on top of the other in the spinal column.

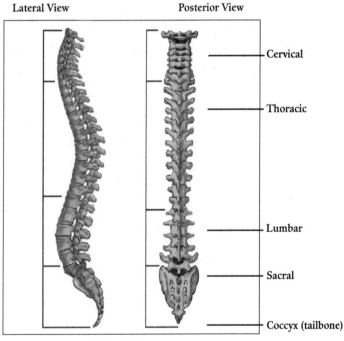

Lateral View   Posterior View

Cervical

Thoracic

Lumbar

Sacral

Coccyx (tailbone)

Spinal Column

Cancellous bone (cancel-lus bone) is a structural component of each vertebra that resembles criss-crossing lattice-work. Its spongy characteristic helps each vertebra to absorb external pressure. The discs are made of dense cartilage that help to absorb and distribute shock and, prevent the vertebrae from grinding together during movement.

The spine has four natural curves. Two curves are **lordotic** (lor-dot-ick, lordosis) and two are **kyphotic** (kye-fah-tick, kyphosis). The **cervical** (sir-ve-kal) and **lumbar** (lum-bar) curves are lordotic. The **thoracic** (thor-as-ick) and **sacral** (say-kral) curves are kyphotic. Each curve serves to distribute mechanical stress.

The atlas, axis, **cervical** spine, thoracic spine, lumbar spine, sacrum (say-krum), and coccyx (cock-six, tailbone) are the bony elements of the spinal column.

The **atlas** and **axis** are the first two cervical vertebrae below the skull. These structures do not look like typical vertebrae. The atlas is ring-shaped; it balances and supports the head. The axis has a tooth-like projection called the **odontoid process** (oh-don-toyed process) that fits up into the atlas. Combined, these two structures enable the head to turn from side-to-side. The atlas pivots around the axis.

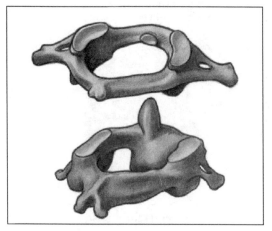

Atlas (top) and Axis (bottom)
© SpineUniverse.com. Used with permission.

Five **cervical** vertebrae are located below the atlas and axis. The **thoracic** spine contains 12 vertebrae and is located in the chest area. The ribs connect to the thoracic spine and protect many organs. Below the thoracic spine is the **lumbar** spine. Although most people have five lumbar vertebrae, it is not unusual to have six. The lumbar vertebrae are the largest and carry most of the body's weight. The **sacrum** and **coccyx** are uniquely shaped.

Medical professionals may abbreviate the levels of the spinal column. For example, the seven cervical vertebrae (including the axis and atlas) are abbreviated C1, C2, C3, C4, C5, C6, and C7. The thoracic levels are T1 through T12 and the lumbar spine is referred to as L1-L5 (or L6). The sacrum is S1 and the coccyx is not abbreviated or numbered.

Each vertebra is separated by an **intervertebral disc.** A disc is made of **fibrocartilage** (fybro-car-til-ledge); a type of cartilage composed of a dense matrix of **collagen** fibers giving the disc great tensile strength. Discs function to absorb and distribute shock from movement and prevent each vertebra from grinding against the other.

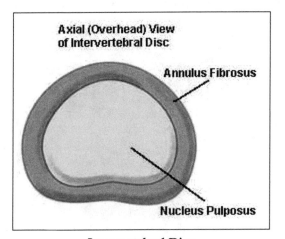

Intervertebral Disc

A disc is similar to a doughnut with jelly filling. The outer ring-shaped area of the disc is called the **annulus fibrosus** (an-you-lus fye-bro-sis). The inner filling is the **nucleus pulposus** (new-klee-us pul-poe-sis). The annulus fibrosus is composed of strong circular layers of **fibrocartilage** that encase the nucleus pulposus; an elastic gel-like substance. **Endplates,** made of fibrocartilage firmly hold each intervertebral disc between the upper and lower vertebrae.

Facet joints (fah-set joints) are also called **zygapophyseal joints** (zye-gap-o-fiz-e-all joints). The joints are located at the posterior (rear) of the cervical, thoracic and lumbar spine. Each facet joint enables movement. Two vertebrae form a pair of facet joints. The facets from the upper and lower vertebrae join together—similar to entwined fingers to form a facet joint. Like other joints in the body, the articulating (ar-tick-you-lating) or moving surfaces are coated with smooth cartilage to facilitate easy movement.

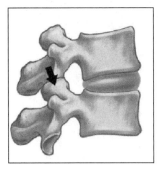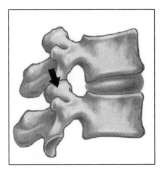

Facet Joints in Motion

© SpineUniverse.com. Used with permission.

The **spinal cord, nerve roots** and brain make up the **Central Nervous System (CNS).** The spinal cord is a flexible cable about 18-inches long and three-quarter's of an inch thick. It is the core of the communication system between the brain and the body. The vertebrae, three membranes called **meninges** (men-in-jez), and **cerebrospinal fluid (CSF)** (sir-ee-bro-spinal fluid) protect the spinal cord.

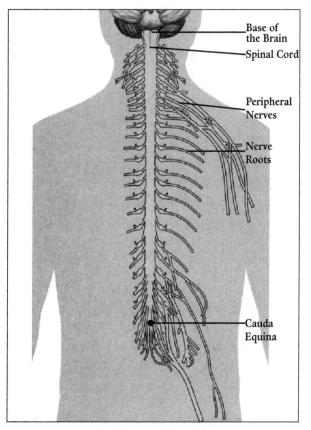

Spinal Nerve Structures
© SpineUniverse.com. Used with permission.

Vertebral arches (ver-tee-brawl arches) are naturally formed at the rear or posterior section of each vertebral body. These arches create a protective hollow canal where the spinal cord is located.

The **dura mater** (doo-rah matter), **arachnoid membrane** (ah-rack-noid membrane) and the **pia mater** (pee-ah-matter) are the three protective meninges (men-in-jez) surrounding the spinal cord. The dura mater is the tough outer layer and the arachnoid is a web-like membrane that attaches to the pia mater; a thin membrane closest to the spinal cord. **Cerebrospinal fluid (CSF)** circulates around and cushions the spinal cord.

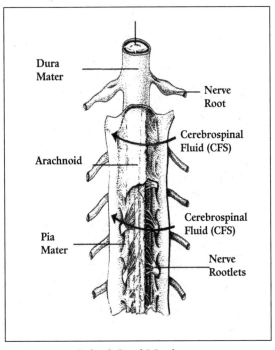

Spinal Cord Meninges

© SpineUniverse.com. Used with permission.

There is 31-pair of spinal **nerve root** fibers that shoot off from the spinal cord similar to tree branches. Each nerve root exits the spinal canal through a **vertebral foramen** (foe-ray-men), also called the **neuroforamen** (nu-row for-a-men). The vertebral foramen are pathways for nerve roots that are naturally created between an upper and lower vertebra. The vertebral foramen are located on the left and right sides of the intervertebral disc. The nerves beyond each spinal nerve root branch outward throughout the body to form thousands of nerve pathways that make up the **Peripheral Nervous System (PNS)**.

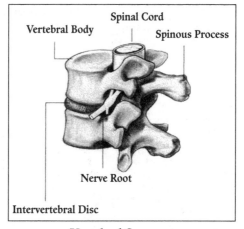

Vertebral Segment

The spinal cord ends near the first lumbar vertebrae (L1). Thereafter begins a nerve structure called the **cauda equina** (caw-dah e-kwhy-nah), which resembles the tail of a horse.

Ligaments (lig-ah-ments) connect bone to bone and tendons attach muscle to bone. Ligaments and **tendons** are fibrous connective tissues composed of densely packed collagen fibers. The blood supply to these tissues is limited and therefore injured ligaments and tendons may take a long time to heal.

Spinal ligaments help provide structural stability. The two primary ligament systems in the spine are the **intrasegmental** and **intersegmental**. The intrasegmental system holds individual vertebrae together and includes the **ligamentum flavum** (lig-ah-mentum flay-vum), **interspinous** (in-ter-spy-nus) and **intertransverse** (in-ter-tranz-verse) ligaments. The intersegmental system holds many vertebrae together and includes the anterior (an-tear-e-or) and **posterior** (pose-tear-e-or) **longitudinal ligaments** and the **supraspinous** (sue-pra-spine-us) ligaments.

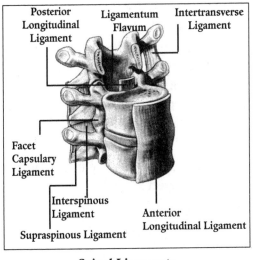

Spinal Ligaments
© SpineUniverse.com. Used with permission.

More than 30 **muscles** and **tendons** (ten-duns) help to provide spinal balance, stability, and mobility. Usually working in groups, muscles contract and relax in response to nerve impulses that originate in the brain. Nerve impulses travel to and from the brain through the spinal cord to and from a specific location in the body via the peripheral nervous system.

The types of **vertebral muscle** include forward flexors, lateral flexors, rotators, and extensors. These different types of muscle groups allow the body to bend forward, side-to-side, twist and bend backward. Muscle is the only type of body tissue with the ability to contract. Muscle shortens and thickens during contraction. When muscle contracts the opposing muscle relaxes. Together—muscles, tendons and ligaments support the spine, hold it upright, and control movement during rest and activity.

Layers of fibrous connective tissue called **fascia** (fay-sha) cover muscles. Fascia extends beyond the muscle to become the tendon that attaches the muscle to bone.

An elaborate system of arteries and veins make up the spine's

vascular system (blood supply). Circulation nourishes cells in the vertebrae, spinal cord, nerves, muscles and other structures. Spinal cells need plasma to reproduce and repair damage. Red blood carries oxygen to cells (e.g. muscle) to burn glucose for energy. White blood cells provide immunity and help to fight infection. A healthy vascular system is necessary to heal an injury and to fight disease.

Conclusion

It is not necessary to know the name of each muscle, nerve or vein in the spine. It is important to be able to identify the basic structures. Equipped with this information, readers are helped to better understand the chapters about spinal disorders and treatments presented in this book.

4

Spinal Disorders

Spinal Disorders: A Synopsis

Stewart G. Eidelson, MD

There are many causes of back and neck pain. Aging, injury, hereditary factors and lifestyle impact the well-being of the spine. Although there is no 'magic bullet' to halt aging, great strides have been made in medicine and the health sciences to increase longevity and quality of life. Sometimes though, despite efforts to keep body weight in check, exercise, and work toward a healthy lifestyle, a spinal problem develops. There are several types of spinal problems including soft tissue and structural disorders and those of a degenerative or congenital (at birth) nature.

Part 1: Soft Tissue Disorders— Muscles, Tendons, Ligaments

Sprains and **strains** are common overuse injuries meaning a muscle, tendon or ligament has been forced to move beyond its normal range of motion. Symptoms include sudden, sharp or persistent pain at the injury site followed by swelling. The pain can be so severe that the patient may fear a bone has broken. Most sprains/strains are not serious and self-heal within two to three weeks.

Anatomically, the bulk of the back is muscle—the spine's work-horses. Regular exercise helps to strengthen muscles enabling them to work harder longer. The **tendons** and **ligaments** may be involved in a sprain/strain type of injury. Tendons attach muscle to bone and ligaments attach bone to bone.

Besides injury caused by overuse, accidents can cause sprain/ strain too. For example, during a motor vehicle accident the body may be suddenly and forcefully thrown forward, backward, and sideways. These movements can cause the muscles, tendons, and ligaments to hyperextend (excessive forward movement) and hyper- flex (excessive backward movement). **Hyperextension** (hi-per ex- ten-shun) and **hyperflexion** (hi-per-flex-un) can cause soft tissues to stretch or tear.

A spinal sprain/strain can be painful and temporarily disabling and this is why a patient often seeks medical attention. The treating physician may include an x-ray in the examination to rule out frac- ture. Typical treatment includes medication to ease pain and relieve **muscle spasm** and **inflammation** (in-flah-may-shun). The treat- ment plan may include a course of physical therapy accompanied by a stretching program.

A stretching program under the guidance of a physical therapist **(physical therapy)** can help prevent the formation of scar tissue, which can be debilitating. Scar tissue is not normal tissue but tissue that forms as part of the natural healing process. The physical ther- apist may be able to train the scar tissue to mimic the function of normal tissue by providing some limited strength.

Muscle spasms occur when a muscle is overworked or over- stretched. The spasm is the response to the injury. Muscle spasms are common and the pain can be intense and disabling. Sometimes the severity of the spasm affects the patient's posture; for example making it difficult to stand up straight.

Whiplash is a **hyperextension** and **hyperflexion** injury that causes micro-trauma to the soft tissues in the neck and upper back. The pain may radiate from the neck into the shoulders, arms and hands. Other symptoms include headache, numbness, tingling, weakness, or burning sensations. Treatment may include a prescription for a soft cervical collar that the patient wears to immobilize the neck and lift the weight of the skull off tender neck, shoulder and upper back tissues. In most cases, whiplash heals in four to six weeks. Rarely does whiplash cause a severe disorder that requires spine surgery.

Part 2: Soft Tissue Disorders: Spinal Nerves

Compressive Neuropathy (compressive ner-row-path-ee) means nerve compression and can affect any nerve in the body. In the spine, a compressive neuropathy refers to the spinal nerves such as the **nerve roots**. The nerve roots exit the spinal canal through the **neuroforamen** (nu-row for-a-men); the pathways for nerve roots naturally created between each upper and lower vertebra. If any of these special nerve passageways become narrowed or clogged, the spinal nerve is compressed and reacts by swelling and causing pain. This disorder is called **foraminal stenosis** (foe-ray-min-al sten-oh-sis) and is a type of compressive neuropathy. Foraminal refers to the neuroforamen and stenosis means narrowing of a passageway.

Bone spurs and disc disorders including a 'slipped', ruptured (**herniated**) or **bulging disc** may displace a spinal nerve causing compression. A compressive neuropathy can cause pain to **radiate** (ray-dee-ate) from the spine down into the buttocks, legs and into the feet. Other symptoms such as tingling, numbness and weakness may accompany pain. In the lumbar spine and lower extremity these symptoms are characterized as '**sciatica**' (sy-attic-ka).

Sciatica (sy-attic-ka) is not a disorder but a symptom of a **compressive neuropathy** (compressive ner-row-path-ee) that may involve the lumbar spinal nerves and the sciatic nerve. The sciatic nerve is the longest and largest nerve in the body. The sciatic nerve begins near the buttocks. As the main sciatic nerve travels downward toward the legs, branches of the main nerve innervate muscles in the lower extremities.

31

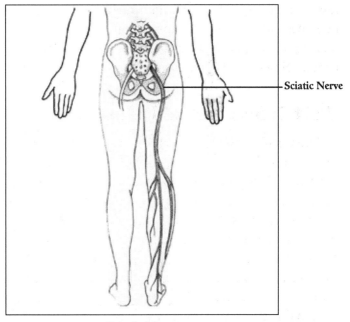

Sciatic Nerve

The sciatic nerve can be damaged during a fall or if an intervertebral disc or bone spur compresses the main nerve or its branches. Pain can be intense and disabling. Sciatica is usually treated without surgery by means of medication and steroid injections to alleviate pain and calm inflammation. In rare circumstances, the cause (e.g. **herniated disc**) of nerve compression may create the need for surgical intervention.

Peripheral Neuropathy (pe-rif-er-al nu-rop-ah-thee) is a degenerative, toxic or nutritional condition affecting the nerves that branch into the body's extremities—the arms, hands, legs and feet. Diabetes or certain drugs can cause peripheral neuropathy. The disease causes the peripheral or distant part of the nerves to shrink and deteriorate to the point that nerves are no longer able to carry impulses. Sensory (feeling) and motor (movement) function may be lost. Symptoms include burning, pins and needles sensation, numbness in the toes or fingers, and weakness in grip or while walking. Prescription medications may help to slow the affects of peripheral neuropathy but may not cure or stop its progression.

Part 3: Soft Tissue Disorders: Infections

Spinal Infections are rare and usually painful. Immediate medical attention is necessary. Untreated, a spinal infection may cause permanent injury or take root in the epidural space; a fatty area adjacent to the spinal nerve roots. **Epidural spaces** (ep-e-do-ral spaces) (or cavities) are found in the cervical, thoracic and lumbar spine. A diagnosis of spinal infection is usually confirmed by MRI. Non-surgical treatment may include intravenous or oral antibiotics combined with best rest. In some cases, surgical intervention may be necessary to eradicate the infection.

Spinal Meningitis (spinal men-in-ji-tis) is an infection causing the membranes in the brain and spinal cord to swell. Symptoms often include fever, weakness, radiating pain, muscle spasms, sensitivity to touch, decreased spinal flexibility, fatigue, sweats, and weight loss. When a child has spinal meningitis, symptoms may include refusal to stand or sit due to pain. In older children and adults increased backache may indicate spinal meningitis. Neck pain and sensitivity to light are common symptoms. This is a serious disease that may require hospitalization. Treatment usually includes intravenous or oral antibiotics combined with bed rest.

Part 4: Structural Disorders: Spinal Fractures

A **Compression Fracture** is a common type of spinal fracture that can involve one or more vertebrae. When an external force exceeds the strength of a vertebral body, the bone collapses. This may cause the front part of the vertebral body to crush forming a wedge shape. Sometimes compression fractures are called **Wedge Fractures.** If the vertebral body breaks apart, then the fracture is called a **Burst Fracture.** X-ray is performed to determine the type of fracture.

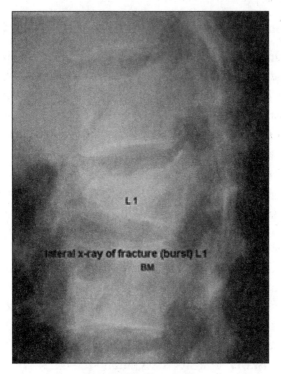

L 1

lateral x-ray of fracture (burst) L 1
BM

X-Ray (Radiograph)
Lateral (side) image of a vertebral burst fracture.
© SpineUniverse.com. Used with permission.

A **burst fracture** is a typical example of an 'unstable' fracture. This means that one or more parts of the broken bone may drift or become pressed against soft tissues, such as the spinal cord or nerve structures. In general, any type of spinal fracture is considered serious and requires immediate medical attention.

Besides the vertebrae, other bony structures serve as protective armor that encases the spinal cord and 31 pair of nerve roots. Other bony spinal structures susceptible to fracture include the **facet joints** (fah-set joints), **pars articularis** (parz are-tick-you-lar-es), and spinous processes. Causes of spinal fracture include trauma, tumors, and **osteoporosis** (os-t-o-pour-o-sis).

Pain is the most prominent symptom of a spinal fracture. Neurological symptoms include tingling, numbness, weakness, and difficulty with balance or when walking. **Compression fractures** that occur in the upper back may cause 'humpback', sometimes a characteristic of **osteoporosis**.

Osteoporosis is the foremost cause of **Compression Fractures.** It is a metabolic disease that robs the bones of nutrients necessary to stay dense and strong. Bones affected by osteoporosis become porous, weak, and sometimes delicate as porcelain. A **Bone Mineral Density** test can help to prevent osteoporosis by detecting low bone mass early.

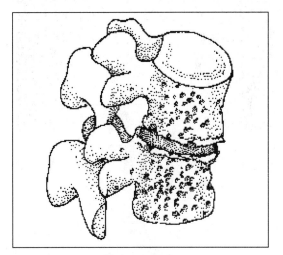

Osteoporosis

35

One of the body's first responses to fracture is to begin healing. The first step involves the formation of a **callus** (cal-us) made up of granular material at the fracture site. A protein, **collagen** (call-ah-gin) is transported to the injury site via the blood stream and works to mend and knit the bone together. As new bone is made it is joined with the old and hardened by means of a process called **calcification** (kals-see-fi-cay-shun).

Treatment usually includes pain medication and bracing. **Braces** are custom-fitted, removable, and designed for comfort. Fortunately, most spinal fractures do not require surgical intervention. In cases of painful compression fractures, new procedures such as **Vertebroplasty** (ver-tee-bro-plasty) and **Kyphoplasty** (kye-foe-plasty) can help to restore the vertebral body and relieve pain.

Spondylolisthesis (spon-de-low-lis-thee-sis) is a disorder where one vertebra in the spine slips over the one below. This disorder most commonly affects the lumbar vertebrae. The severity of a spondylolisthesis is determined using a standardized grading system. Grade 1 is the least advanced and means that 25% of the vertebra has slipped forward over the vertebra below it. Grade 5 is the most advanced and means the vertebra has completely slid forward and over the vertebra below.

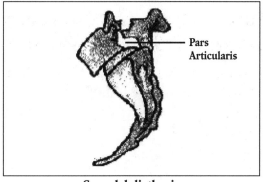

Pars Articularis

Spondylolisthesis

© SpineUniverse.com Used with permission.

There are primarily two types of spondylolisthesis: Developmental or Acquired. Developmental Spondylolisthesis may be congenital (present at birth) or discovered later in life. During childhood, if the **pars articularis** (parz are-tick-you-lar-es) does not fuse during early development, a structural weakness is created. This can make the spine susceptible to a spondylolisthesis later in life. Acquired Spondylolisthesis develops from daily wear and tear, degenerative changes in the spine or trauma.

Some patients are symptom free and learn that they have a spondylolisthesis after an x-ray for a different problem. Typical symptoms include low back pain (especially after activity), thigh or leg pain, swayback, and walking that resembles waddling.

In most cases, spondylolisthesis requires no treatment or is treated non-surgically. The spine specialist may prescribe or suggest over-the-counter medications to treat pain and inflammation. Sometimes steroid injections into the spine are helpful to relieve symptoms. The use of a brace may be prescribed to support the spine and relieve muscle spasm and pain. Patients with spondylolisthesis are advised to avoid activities that stress the lumbar spine such as weightlifting, football, and gymnastics. Seldom is surgery necessary.

Part 5: Structural Disorders: Abnormal Spinal Curvature

Scoliosis (sko-lee-oh-sis) is a term taken from a Greek word that means curvature. The disease causes the spine to curve laterally (to the side) into the shape of an 'S' or 'C'. The visible physical signs include uneven shoulders or hips and a rib hump when the patient bends forward at the waist.

During the 19th Century physicians thought that poor posture was the primary cause of scoliosis. However, today it is known that scoliosis can be congenital (present at birth) or caused by neuromuscular disorders such as cerebral palsy or from degenerative changes such as those resulting from the collapse of vertebral bodies. Another type of scoliosis is **Idiopathic Scoliosis** (id-dee-oh-path-ick sko-lee-oh-sis). The term 'idiopathic' means the cause is unknown, although there is a strong hereditary factor with idiopathic scoliosis.

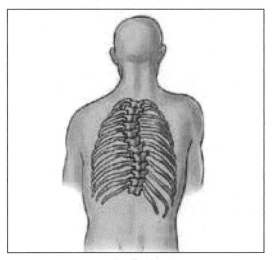

Scoliosis

© SpineUniverse.com. Used with permission.

Most cases are found during scoliosis screening at school, by the family physician, or when the child wears a swim suit. A full-length x-ray of the spine is ordered to determine the size and severity of the curve. Further, the x-ray is used to measure the degree of curvature.

Bracing is the standard treatment choice to help stabilize a curve from progressing. In adolescent patients, the curve may stabilize as maturity is reached. Periodic x-ray studies are ordered to monitor the curve. Surgery is a consideration if the curve is severe and progressive.

Kyphosis (kye-foe-sis) is the normal curvature of the thoracic spine (chest, rib cage). However, excessive or abnormal kyphosis may develop from poor posture or **osteoporosis** (os-t-o-pour-o-sis). Patients with abnormal kyphosis appear bent over or may be humpback.

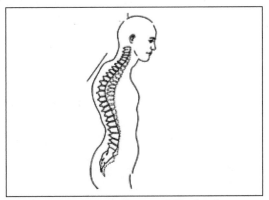

Excessive or abnormal Kyphosis

Lordosis (lor-doe-sis) is the normal curve found in the neck and low back. When lordosis is excessive, such as in some patients with **spondylolisthesis** (spon-de-low-lis-thee-sis), the low back appears as swayback.

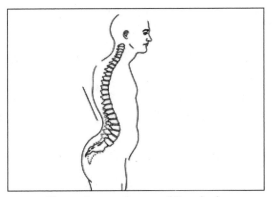

Excessive or abnormal Lordosis

Part 6: Disorders Affecting Intervertebral Discs

The intervertebral discs act as shock-absorbing cushions between the vertebrae. Although some people use the term **Slipped Disc** to denote a disc disorder, discs do not slip. In fact, each disc is held firmly in place between two vertebral bodies by **endplates** and a system of spinal **ligaments** (lig-ah-ments).

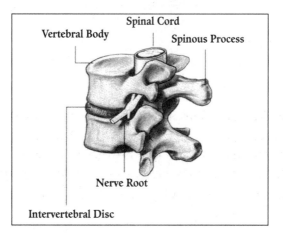

Endplates affix the Intervertebral Disc between the upper and lower vertebrae.

© SpineUniverse.com. Used with permission.

Disc disorders can result from simple activity, excessive spinal strain, poor body mechanics, and the biochemical and degenerative changes that occur during aging. Basically there are two types of disc disorders—characterized as either **Contained** or **Non-Contained.**

A **Bulging Disc** is an example of a **contained** disc disorder. A bulging disc has not broken open; the **nucleus pulposus** (new-klee-us pul-poe-sis) remains contained within the **annulus**

fibrosus (an-you-lus fye-bro-sis). A small bubble-like structure may pop outward from the disc into the spinal canal or onto nerve roots. The gel-like nucleus does not leak out from the disc. A bulging disc could be compared to a volcano prior to eruption and can be a precursor to herniation.

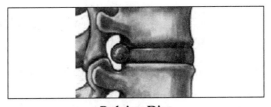

Bulging Disc

© SpineUniverse.com. Used with permission.

A **Non-Contained Disc** is one that has either partially or completely broken open such as a **Herniated Disc** (her-knee-ate-ed disc), or ruptured disc. When a disc herniates, some of the gel-like nucleus leaks outward into the spinal canal and onto nerve structures. The nuclear material contains a chemical irritant that causes inflammation and pain.

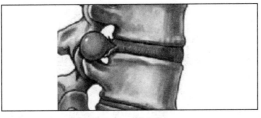

Herniated Disc

© SpineUniverse.com. Used with permission.

A **bulging** or **herniated disc** (her-knee-ate-ed disc) can occur at any level of the spine. Some people are symptom free while others complain of pain, numbness, tingling sensations, or weakness.

Further, symptoms caused by nerve compression may extend or **radiate** (ray-de-ate) into the arms (cervical) or legs (lumbar).

A non-surgical multidisciplinary approach to symptom relief includes pain medication, anti-inflammatory drugs, muscle relaxants, physical therapy, and epidural steroid injections. Seldom is surgical intervention necessary.

Part 7: Degenerative Disorders

Not unlike a mechanical device, the human body is subject to the affects from aging and wear and tear. As the body ages, subtle biochemical changes begin to affect the spine. Degenerative spinal disorders take years to develop and may be associated with past injury, abuse, body structure, congenital problems, or heredity. Many of the more common degenerative spinal disorders are presented below.

Arthritis (arth-rye-tis) affects approximately 80% of people over age 55 in the United States. Injury, a weakened immune system, and an inherited predisposition can trigger the onset of arthritis. There are hundreds of types of arthritis that share similar symptoms that include inflammation, joint pain, and progressive deterioration of joint surfaces over time.

Typical problems involve the joints losing their normal contour or shape and fluid build-up with debris floating inside the joint capsule. In the spine, arthritis targets the facet joints (fah-set joints) that enable the body to bend and twist. Part of the problem may involve the body's response to the degenerative effects of arthritis—that being the manufacture of bone to try to stop joint movement. The extra bone the body makes is in the form of **bone spurs** or **bony overgrowths**—medically speaking, **osteophytes** (os-t-o-fights).

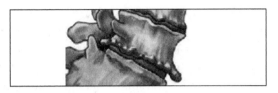

Osteophytes; Bony overgrowths, Bone Spurs
© SpineUniverse.com. Used with permission.

Osteophytes (os-t-o-fight) can be found in areas affected by arthritis such as the joint or disc spaces where **cartilage** (car-til-ledge) has deteriorated. The body's attempt to stop joint movement is really futile as it is never completely successful. The evidence of these bony deposits is found by a standard x-ray study.

When bony overgrowths clog neural passageways where nerve roots leave the spinal canal, nerves become compressed. The result is pain, numbness, and other sensations such as tingling, burning and pins and needles felt in the extremities below the compressed nerve root. Motor symptoms include muscle spasm, cramping, weakness, or loss of muscular control in the affected area of the body.

Osteoarthritis (OA) (os-t-o-arth-rye-tis) is the degenerative form of arthritis. It is a progressive joint disease associated with aging. Many elderly people have some degree of OA in the knees, hips, spine or other joints. Spinal OA affects the **facet joints** (fah-set joints). As the facet joints deteriorate, soft tissues may become inflamed and **cartilage** (car-til-ledge) may begin to fray like an over-used rag. During this process the cartilage begins to break away from the joint surfaces. Cartilage fragments may begin to float in the **synovial fluid** (si-n-vee-al fluid) that lubricates the joint. Instead of joint surfaces gliding against one another, bones grind against one another during movement. Nerve structures in the joint become irritated and inflamed causing pain.

Similar to **arthritis** (arth-rye-tis), OA may trigger the formation of **osteophytes** (os-t-o-fights). As previously mentioned, these bony spurs are the body's way of dealing with the degenerative

43

disease process. In the spine, osteophytes can cause disc space to narrow. When this happens the adjacent intervertebral disc may collapse. When a disc collapses, the disc height is lost affecting the size of the involved **neuroforamen** (nu-row for-a-men). This can lead to nerve compression and impingement **(Spinal Stenosis,** sten-oh-sis).

Rheumatoid Arthritis (RA) (room-ah-toyed arth-rye-tis) is a progressive form of arthritis that can be painfully destructive. RA can cause joint tissues to swell and thicken. Over time the affected joint disintegrates and may lead to deformity. RA often appears during middle age and is more common in women.

Symptoms include fatigue, weakness, loss of appetite, fever, and anemia. Medication helps to relieve inflammation and pain and regular exercise helps to maintain joint function. Passive forms of physical therapy help to increase joint mobility.

Ankylosing Spondylitis (AS) (an-key-low-sing spon-dee-lie-tis) is a chronic progressive inflammatory spinal disease that causes pain and joint stiffness. AS is part of a group of rheumatic diseases called seronegative spondyloarthropathies (cero-negative spon-dee-low-are-throw-op-ath-ez) that share a human antigen (HLA-B27). As the disease progresses the joints fuse together, vertebral endplates are destroyed, and cartilage hardens. Initially, AS may begin as low back pain with stiffness and tenderness in the sacrum. However, AS is known to progressively move into the cervical spine. Sometimes AS is called 'Bamboo Spine' because over time the spine takes on the appearance of bamboo. The progressive nature of AS lead may lead to deformity.

A standard x-ray is used to detect the development of AS. Conservative non-surgical treatment includes non-steroidal anti-inflammatory drugs (NSAIDs) and physical therapy. Most AS patients do not require surgery. Surgery is considered when pain is severe and unrelenting, neurological problems develop, the spine becomes unstable, and deformity affects daily life.

Spinal Stenosis (spinal sten-oh-sis) is the abnormal narrowing of the **neuroforamen** (nu-row for-a-men) or spinal canal that causes nerve or spinal cord compression. When spinal stenosis affects the neuroforamen it is called **Foraminal Stenosis** (foe-ray-min-al sten-oh-sis). Either form of stenosis can affect any level of the spine, but is most often found in the cervical and lumbar spine in people over age 50. Although there may be a genetic predisposition to spinal stenosis, it appears to be caused by aging and spinal 'wear and tear' from daily activities.

The spine changes as the body ages: spinal ligaments (lig-ah-ments) thicken and harden, joints may enlarge, and **osteophytes** (os-t-o-fights) form. Other disorders that affect the neuroforaminal or canal space are **bulging** and **herniated discs** (her-knee-ate-ed discs) or **spondylolisthesis** (spon-de-low-lis-thee-sis). These disorders can cause nerve or spinal cord compression.

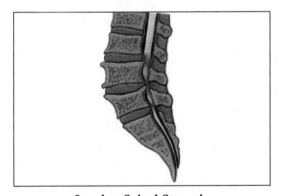

Lumbar Spinal Stenosis
© SpineUniverse.com. Used with permission.

Cervical Spinal Stenosis (sir-ve-kal spinal sten-oh-sis) may cause pain, weakness, or numbness in the shoulders, arms and legs. Hand movements may become clumsy and problems with balance and walking can develop.

Lumbar Spinal Stenosis (lum-bar spinal sten-oh-sis) may cause pain, weakness, or numbness in the legs, calves or buttocks.

It is common for symptoms to increase when walking and decrease when the patient bends forward or sits down. The pain can be severe and radiate (ray-dee-ate) like **sciatica** (sy-attic-ka).

A CT Scan or MRI may be used to confirm the diagnosis. Conservative non-operative treatments to relieve symptoms include NSAIDs, analgesics, **epidural** steroid injections, and **physical therapy**. Surgery may be considered if symptoms become severe or if neurological problems develop (e.g. bladder/bowel dysfunction). The goal of surgery is to relieve spinal cord or nerve compression by enlarging or widening the space. Surgery may involve removing and trimming away parts (e.g. herniated disc) that create pressure.

Degenerative Disc Disease (DDD) is a condition that develops gradually, is associated with the aging process, and affects the structural integrity of the intervertebral discs. The aging process causes biochemical changes throughout the entire body. In the spine these degenerative changes cause discs to dehydrate and weaken. In turn, as discs shrink or flatten, normal disc height is lost affecting the size of the **neuroforamen** (nu-row for-a-men).

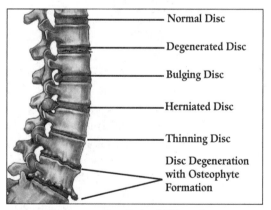

Degenerative Spinal Disorders

© SpineUniverse.com. Used with permission.

46

Although DDD can affect any level of the spine, the lumbar spine is the most common area of reported problems. This is because the lumbar spine carries a large portion of the body's weight and when discs degenerate, their ability to handle mechanical stress decreases.

Degenerative Disc Disease (DDD) can lead to other spinal disorders including **bulging** or **herniated discs** (her-knee-ate-ed discs), **spinal stenosis** (spinal sten-oh-sis), and **spondylolisthesis** (spon-de-low-lis-thee-sis). The narrowing of the disc spaces between the vertebral bodies can be seen on x-ray.

Osteoporosis (os-t-o-pour-o-sis) is known as the silent degenerative disease and is so labeled because during the early stages the patient may be symptom free. The disease causes bones to lose density and strength making them highly susceptible to fracture. In the spine, compression fractures are commonly associated with osteoporosis.

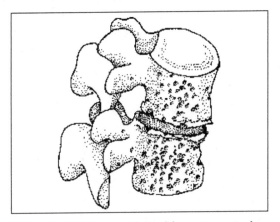

Vertebral bodies weakened by osteoporosis.

Symptoms of **osteoporosis** (os-t-o-pour-o-sis) include chronic pain, muscle spasm, neurological problems, loss of mobility, and an altered appearance. Patients may look frail, bent over, shorter, and deformed with a humpback. Daily activities such as making the bed, removing food from the oven, or even embracing a loved one can cause spontaneous vertebral compression or crush fractures. If the disease is allowed to progress, without proper treatment, the patient's general health may deteriorate.

Men and women are at risk for osteoporosis. Certain lifestyle habits increase the risk and include smoking, alcoholism, heavy laxative use, stress, diabetes, menopause, inactivity, and unhealthy dieting. Women who smoke produce lower levels of estrogen and smoking interferes with calcium absorption necessary for building and maintaining strong bones. Men or women who are alcoholics usually have less bone mass because calcium absorption is hindered. Stress may be an undermining factor because it can stimulate adrenal hormone production causing calcium to pass during urination.

Women tend to be prone to osteoporosis because their bones are smaller and contain less mass. Further, during menopause estrogen levels are affected and estrogen helps to maintain sufficient calcium needed for healthy bones. Plus—women usually live longer than men and therefore have more time to develop osteoporosis.

Osteoporosis (os-t-o-pour-o-sis) is one of the most common bone diseases and can be prevented by early detection combined with a proper diet, program to quit smoking, exercise, supplements, and drug therapies. Osteoporosis can affect the spine, hips, wrists, and other bones in the body.

A simple and quick **Bone Mineral Density** test or **CT Scan** is used to detect osteoporosis early — years before damage control become necessary. Unfortunately, if osteoporosis is not detected early, the disease can ravage the structural integrity of the vertebral bodies leaving bones in a critically weakened state.

Part 8: Spinal Tumors

Spinal Tumors are rare. There are many types of spinal tumors; **benign** (be-nine, non-cancerous) and **malignant** (mal-eg-nant, cancerous). It is rare for a tumor to originate in the spine. These are called **Primary Tumors**. Tumors that spread from one place to another are called **Secondary Tumors** or **Metastatic Tumors**. These tumors are malignant and originated someplace outside of the spine (e.g. breast). The severity of the malignant tumor is graded or scored. The type of tumor, its location and 'score' (unless benign) helps the spine specialist determine how to treat the tumor.

Constant back pain that is not relieved by rest or lying down is the primary symptom of a spinal tumor. Of course, there are many other spinal disorders that share pain as a symptom. Therefore, it is always important to seek medical advice if back pain does not resolve. Other symptoms that could indicate spinal tumor include sciatica, numbness, partial paralysis, spinal deformity, incontinence, and fever. Symptoms usually worsen over time as the tumor grows.

There are several types of imaging tests spine specialists use to diagnose and identify spinal tumors. These tests include x-rays, nuclear bone scan, MRI, and CT Scan. If the imaging study reveals a tumor, the next step is usually a **biopsy** (by-op-see); a sample of the tumor taken during a surgical procedure.

Tumor treatment is dependent on the tumor type, whether it is benign or malignant, its location, and the patient's health. Treatments include chemotherapy, radiation therapy, surgical removal of the tumor, alternative therapies, or a combination of treatments.

Conclusion

Neck and back pain should never be ignored, especially when symptoms are consistent and not relieved by rest. It is wise to search out a spine specialist to treat any of the disorders covered in this chapter.

There are many types of spine specialists including orthopaedic spine surgeons, neurosurgeons, chiropractors, pain management specialists, and physical therapists. Your primary care physician may be a good starting point in your quest for the appropriate treatment.

What is Spinal Stenosis?

Stewart G. Eidelson, MD

The term **spinal stenosis** refers to a disorder that primarily results from the process of growing older. Years ago it was called creeping paralysis. It was accepted that if one got old enough, one could acquire it and have to 'live and die with it'.

The words spinal and stenosis are separated primarily for clarification. **Spinal** denotes the location and stenosis means the condition. **Stenosis** is derived from Greek meaning, narrowing of a normally larger opening. The term stenosis is widely used in medicine for different parts of the body. The primary area discussed here is stenosis of the spine, which can develop in the cervical, thoracic, or lumbar region. We will address the lumbar area in this article because of the greater percentile that we see.

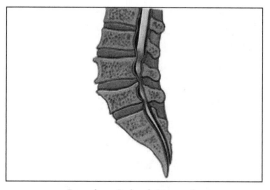

Lumbar Spinal Stenosis

© SpineUniverse.com. Used with permission.

Risk Factors

Factors that predispose a person to developing spinal stenosis can start in the womb as a result of genetics or congenital problems acquired from the mother. In addition, there are many perfectly normal backs that after childhood development are mechanically ruined due to self-destructive modes, but not all self-controlled.

Symptoms can be Debilitating

Eventually the narrowing of the spaces in the spine causes pressure on the spinal cord and/or nerve roots. When the neuroforamina (plural of neuroforamen) are reduced in size due to surrounding debris, the nerves react to the pressure by swelling. As the window closes on the nerve the associated pain may become excruciating and debilitating.

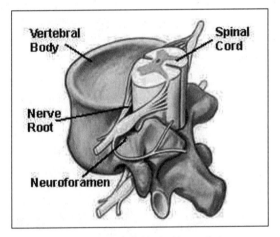

© SpineUniverse.com. Used with permission.

Pain may be felt in the buttocks, thighs, and/or calves when walking and/or standing. Spinal stenosis may also cause numbness, weakness, burning sensations, tingling, and pins and needles in the involved extremity, such as the arm or leg.

Some patients with spinal stenosis may find the pain eases when bending forward or sitting. This may happen because bending forward creates more vertebral space, which may temporarily relieve nerve compression. The doctor may use a variety of approaches to diagnose spinal stenosis and rule out other conditions.

Medical History—the patient tells the doctor details about symptoms and any injury, condition or general health problem that might be causing the symptoms.

Physical Examination—the doctor (1) examines the patient to determine the extent of limitation of movement; (2) checks for pain or symptoms when the patient hyperextends the spine (bends backwards); and (3) looks for the loss of extremity reflexes, which may be related to numbness or weakness in the arm or legs.

X-Ray—an x-ray beam is passed through the back to produce a two-dimensional picture. An x-ray may be done before other tests to look for signs of an injury, tumor, or inherited abnormality. Test results may reveal the structure of the vertebrae, outlines the joints, and can detect calcification.

MRI (Magnetic Resonance Imaging)—energy from a powerful magnet (not x-rays) produces signals that are detected by a scanner and analyzed by a computer. This produces a series of cross-sectional images (slices) and/or a three-dimensional view of parts of the back. A MRI is particularly sensitive for detecting damage or disease of soft tissues, such as the discs between vertebrae or ligaments. It shows the spinal cord, nerve roots, and surrounding spaces, as well as enlargement, degeneration or tumors.

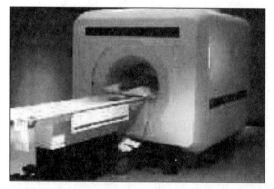

A type of MRI (Magnetic Resonance Imaging) Machine

Computerized Axial Tomography (CAT)—x-rays are passed through the back at different angles, detected by a scanner, and analyzed by a computer. This produces a series of cross-sectional images and/or three-dimensional views of the parts of the back. The scan shows the shape and size of the spinal canal, its contents, and structures surrounding it.

Myelogram—a liquid dye that x-rays cannot penetrate is injected into the spinal column. The dye circulates around the spinal cord and spinal nerves, which appear as white objects against bone on an x-ray film. A myelogram can show pressure on the spinal cord or nerves from herniated discs, bone spurs, or tumors.

Bone Scan—an injected radioactive material attaches itself to bone, especially in areas where bone is actively breaking down or being formed. The test can detect fractures, tumors, infections, and arthritis, but may not tell one disorder from another. Therefore, a bone scan is usually performed along with other tests.

Non-Surgical Treatment

Treatment has improved immensely since the 1950s when the pharmaceutical options were largely limited to aspirin and cortisone. In the absence of severe or progressive nerve involvement, a doctor may prescribe one or more of the following conservative treatments:

1. Non-steroidal anti-inflammatory drugs, such as aspirin, naproxen (Naprosyn®), ibuprofen (Motrin®, Nuprin®, Advil®), to reduce inflammation and relieve pain. New generation Cox-2 inhibitors have shown remarkable results in many cases.
2. Analgesics, such as acetaminophen (Tylenol®), to relieve pain.
3. Corticosteroid injections into the outermost portion of the membranes covering the spinal cord and nerve roots to reduce inflammation and treat acute pain that radiates into the hips or down a leg.

4. Restricted activity (varies depending on extent of nerve involvement).

5. Physical therapy and/or prescribed exercises to maintain motion of the spine and build endurance, which help stabilize the spine.

6. A lumbar brace or corset to provide some support and help the patient regain mobility. This approach is sometimes used with patients with weak abdominal muscles or older patients with degeneration at several levels of the spine.

Spine Surgery

Like all surgeons, I view surgery as the last resort following a complete exploration of other treatment options. You may be surprised to know that fewer than 5% of patients consulting a spine specialist ever actually have surgery. The most common surgical solution to spinal stenosis is a laminectomy. The term is derived from two words: lamina (part of the spinal canal's bony roof) and ectomy (removal).

The object of a laminectomy is to remove the pressure on the nerve root. The pressure is the cause of the pain and other debilitating effects of stenosis. The operation can be performed using traditional or microsurgical techniques. The decision is largely governed by the surgeon's preference. The surgeon removes bone and debris from the foramen to reduce pressure on the nerve root.

Healing and Recovery

Healing is the body's natural process of restoring its damaged tissues to a normal or nearly normal state. Although healing may be improved by general good health, proper nutrition, rest and physical fitness, healing is a natural process.

Recovery is the process during which the patient works to become well. It requires a gradual but persistent effort to increase physical strengths and minimize weaknesses. The patient must concentrate on what is improving, rather than on what symptoms remain. This focus on the progress made, combined with a constant effort to improve, make up the positive attitude that will speed the patient's return to normal daily activity over the next three months.

5

Non-Surgical Treatment

Treating Back and Neck Pain without Surgery

Stewart G. Eidelson, MD

Introduction

Seldom does back pain require surgical intervention. A conservative treatment plan may include bed rest for a day or two combined with medication to reduce inflammation and pain. Medications recommended by the physician are based on the patient's medical condition, age, other drugs the patient currently takes, and safety.

The first choice for pain relief is often nonsteroidal anti-inflammatory drugs (NSAIDs). These drugs should be taken with food to reduce the risk of stomach upset and stomach bleeding. Muscle relaxants may provide relief from muscle spasm but are actually benign sedatives, which often cause drowsiness. Narcotic pain relievers may be prescribed for use during the acute phase.

Part 1: Braces and Traction

A cervical collar may be recommended to help a patient with neck pain. Cervical collars limit movement and support the head taking the load off the neck. Lying down has a similar affect. Limiting neck movement and reducing pressure (weight) gives muscles needed rest while healing.

Cervical traction may be prescribed for home use. This form of traction gently pulls the head, stretching neck muscles, while increasing the size of the neural passageways (foramen). An example of a cervical traction device is presented on the following page.

Neckpro™ Overdoor Cervical (Neck) Traction Device
Chattanooga Group

Neckpro™ is a home over-the-door unit for cervical traction. Cervical traction may be used to relieve neck pain associated with disc herniation, osteoarthritis, cervical radiculopathy (e.g. pinched nerve), fibromyalgia, whiplash, and tension headaches. Further, cervical traction may relieve muscle tension and spasm in the upper back, shoulders, and neck. Cervical traction gently lifts the weight of the head off the neck anatomy and may temporarily decompress pinched and inflamed nerves.

Neckpro™ is unlike conventional over-the-door traction systems that utilize a bag of water. Systems utilizing a bag of water require the patient to undergo a period of trial and error to determine the right amount of water to equal the needed weight for traction to be effective.

Neckpro™ couples a computer designed, precision-made compression spring with a unique ratcheting device that delivers a more precise amount of cervical traction tension. Traction tension is delivered gradually and allows the patient to monitor and keep track of the settings used for the best outcome.

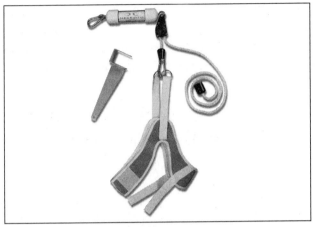

© Chattanooga Group. Used with permission.

The Neckpro™ Overdoor Cervical Traction device is easy to set up. The head halter is comfortable even under high levels of cervical traction tension.

Part 2: Physical Therapy (PT)

PT may be incorporated into the patient's treatment plan once activity can be tolerated. PT may include ice therapy to slow nerve conduction thereby decreasing inflammation and pain. Heat treatments may be used to accelerate soft tissue repair. Heat increases blood flow and speeds up the metabolic rate to assist healing. Heat also helps decrease muscle spasm, pain, and promotes a relaxed feeling.

A type of moist heating pad is featured on the following page.

TheraTherm® Digital Moist Heating Pad
Chattanooga Group

Moist heat is a common therapy used to temporarily relieve muscle spasm and inflammation caused by strain and tension. The

TheraTherm® Digital heating pad is designed for home use and is easy to use.

The TheraTherm® product draws moisture from the air and holds it in a specially designed flannel cover. Moisture is rapidly heated by high-grade ceramics that allow deeper penetration of heat into the body's soft tissues.

The digital hand control allows the patient to select a temperature between 88- and 166-degrees Fahrenheit and treatment time between 1 to 60 minutes.

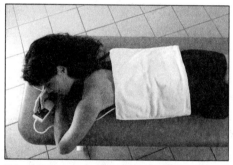

**TheraTherm® Digital moist heating pad
can be used to ease low back pain.**

© Chattanooga Group. Used with permission.

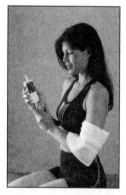

TheraTherm® can be used to soothe stiff joints.

© Chattanooga Group. Used with permission.

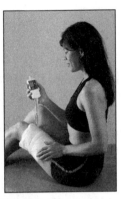

TheraTherm® can be used to calm sore leg muscles.

© Chattanooga Group. Used with permission.

Ultrasound is a treatment used to deliver heat deep into soft tissues. Sometimes a heat treatment is given prior to a session of therapeutic exercise.

Therapeutic exercise can help build strength, increase range of motion, coordination, stability, balance, and promotes relaxation. Therapists educate their patients about their condition and teach posture correction and relaxation techniques. Patients who participate in a structured physical therapy program often progress to wellness more rapidly than those who do not. This includes back maintenance through a home exercise program developed for the patient by the physical therapist.

Neck and back pain is extremely common in today's society. More than 65 million Americans suffer from back pain every year. In fact, back pain is the most common reason why people seek medical care.

Thanks to medical advances and technology there are now numerous treatment options for people who suffer from back and neck pain. But, just as each patient is an individual, not all options are available or appropriate for everyone. If you are a back pain sufferer, talk to your doctor about which treatment options are best for you. The following is a brief discussion about the most commonly used treatments for back pain available today.

Part 3: Drug Therapies

Today, patients have a wide variety of medications to choose from to treat their back pain. Some drugs not only relieve pain but also work to reduce inflammation and relax muscle tension and spasm. However, many of these medications, even those available without a prescription, can have serious side effects. Talk to your doctor before taking any medications for back pain.

Non-Steroidal Anti-Inflammatory Drugs (NSAIDs) include aspirin, ibuprofen, Naproxen®, Ketoprofen® and many more. Anti-inflammatory medications help reduce swelling and inflammation and promote healing. When taken in low doses, NSAIDs work as mild analgesics. When taken in higher doses and on a regular basis, enough of the drug builds up to have a true anti-inflammatory effect.

COX-2 Inhibitors are a type of NSAID and include celecoxib (brand name Celebrex®). These medications, approved by the Food and Drug Administration (FDA), allow patients to take higher doses without the accompanying gastrointestinal side effects from conventional NSAIDs.

Acetaminophen such as Tylenol®, Anacin-3®, Phenaphen®, Valadol®, and other brands are analgesics. Analgesic medications are used to treat acute or some forms of chronic pain. They are the most common alternatives to NSAIDs. Acetaminophen can be used alone or in combination with NSAIDs. Liver and kidney damage are potential serious side effects of acetaminophen use.

Opioids such as morphine and codeine, meperidine (Demerol®), or oxycodone-release (Oxycontin®) are rarely used and only if pain is severe. Due to their addictive nature, these drugs are not routinely prescribed, as some physicians believe they do more harm than good.

Muscle Relaxants such as cyclobenzaprine (Flexeril®), diazepam (Valium®), carisoprodol (Soma®), or methocarbamol (Robaxin®) are often prescribed for severe pain. However, some experts believe that NSAIDs are just as effective.

Part 4: Spinal Injections

With most spinal injections, a local anesthetic called Lidocaine (also known as Xylocaine®) is used to numb the injection site. A steroid medication called a corticosteroid is also commonly injected along with the anesthetic in order to reduce inflammation in the affected areas.

Facet Joint Injection

When back pain originates from the facet joints (located on each side of the vertebrae), a specific type of injection called a facet joint injection may reduce inflammation and provide pain relief. Doctors use fluoroscopy to ensure the needle is correctly placed before the medicines are injected. Fluoroscopy is a special type of x-ray used to project live images onto a monitor (TV screen).

Epidural Steroid Injection (ESI)

During an ESI, medications are injected into the 'epidural space'. The epidural space is the area between the spinal sac and spinal canal, which runs the length of the canal. As the medicine is injected into the epidural space it coats the nerve roots and outside lining of the facet joints.

Part 5: Other Non-Surgical Treatments
Stewart G. Eidelson, MD

Acupuncture

Acupuncture is one of the oldest, most commonly used alternative or 'complimentary medical' procedures in the world. Originating in China more than 2,000 years ago, acupuncture became widely known in the United States in the 1970s. Studies have documented acupuncture's effects, but they have not been able to fully explain how acupuncture works.

Lifestyle, age, physiology and other factors combine to make every person different. A treatment that works for one person may not work for another who has the same condition. You, as a health care consumer (especially if you have a pre-existing medical condition) should discuss acupuncture with your doctor. Do not rely on a diagnosis of disease by an acupuncturist who does not have substantial conventional medical training. If you have received a diagnosis from a doctor and have had little or no success using conventional medicine, you may wish to ask your doctor whether acupuncture might help.

Chiropractic

Chiropractic is a branch of the healing arts based on the understanding that good health depends, in part, upon a normally functioning nervous system. The spinal column is a key structure in the nervous system as it contains the spinal cord and nerve roots that branch out into the entire body. Chiropractors do not prescribe drugs or perform surgery. Chiropractic treatment involves adjusting the spine to correct vertebral misalignment and imbalance.

Pain Management

Pain management is an important part of health care directed at alleviating or reducing acute, chronic, and cancer pain. Pain management generally includes anesthesiology, physiatry, and physical medicine and rehabilitation. The types of treatment offered by a pain management specialist include, but are not limited to analgesics, narcotics, anti-depressants, biofeedback, epidural injections, nerve blocks, transcutaneous electric nerve stimulation (TENs), and spinal cord stimulation.

Physical Therapy (PT)

The treating doctor prescribes PT to treat sprains/strains, muscles spasms, arthritis, and many other neck and back disorders. It is an important component of treatment following spine surgery. The purpose of PT is to help the patient build strength, flexibility, and endurance. PT combines treatments such as heat/cold therapy, ultrasound, electrical stimulation, and massage with exercise as part of rehabilitation.

Conclusion

The relationship you have with your doctor is important. He (or she) will work to diagnose the cause of your back pain. A proper diagnosis is the first step to develop the right treatment plan for you.

Intelect® Portable Electrotherapy
Chattanooga Group

Electrotherapy, or electrical stimulation as it is often called, is believed to block the transmission of pain signals along nerves. The therapy promotes the release of the body's natural painkillers, endorphins. Electrical stimulation is used to increase local blood circulation, relax muscle spasms, prevent or retard muscle atrophy, and maintain or increase range of motion.

Electrotherapy is administered using a device called a TENS unit. TENS is the acronym for transcutaneous (through the skin) electrical nerve stimulators. A TENS device delivers low-frequency electrical current through electrode patches placed on the skin over the painful area (e.g. low back).

Pictured following are two TENS devices from the Intelect® line of portable high-volt electrotherapy units. The Intelect® units allow the patient to adjust the intensity of the current, select continuous or pulsed, and set the desired duration of therapy.

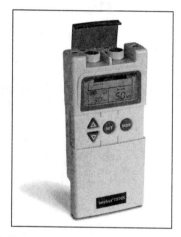

© Chattanooga Group. Used with permission.

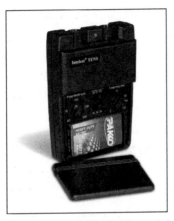

© Chattanooga Group. Used with permission.

Therapeutic Spinal Traction
Susan A. Spinasanta

Mechanical and Compressive Pain

There are many types of disorders known to cause back pain including those defined as mechanical and/or compressive. Mechanical back pain commonly stems from injury or a degenerative process affecting discs, joints, ligaments and/or muscles. Pain from an irritated or 'compressed' nerve root, such as in sciatica (sy-attic-ka), is termed compressive pain.

Conservative forms of treatment may include non-steroidal anti-inflammatory medication, a muscle relaxant, a prescription drug for pain during the acute phase, and physical therapy. Along with these therapies, spinal traction may be recommended.

Spinal Traction—What It Does

Therapeutic spinal traction uses manually or mechanically created forces to stretch and mobilize the spine. Traction may alleviate back pain by stretching tight spinal muscles that result from spasm and widen intervertebral foramen (foe-ray-men) to relieve nerve root impingement.

Patient Evaluation

Each patient is unique and what works well for one patient may not be appropriate for another. Therefore, each prospective patient is carefully evaluated prior to treatment. This assessment enables the therapist to make decisions about the type of traction to be utilized, the force/weight of distraction, and the duration of treatment.

The goal of traction is to reduce pain to assist the patient to become more functional. Therapy should be relaxing—not cause additional or new pain. Therefore, the initial session of therapeutic traction typically uses less force or weight during distraction (pull away). The therapist carefully follows cues from the patient relative to their tolerance level, which includes bodily positioning.

Traction Techniques

Techniques applied in spinal traction are dependent in part on the patient's physical condition, disorder, individual tolerance, and the spinal level(s) to be treated. Application of traction may be manual, positional, or mechanical. Traction may be applied as a continuous force or intermittently. The techniques presented below are not all inclusive.

Cervical Traction

Manual therapeutic traction is a hands-on approach. The patient lies in a relaxed and comfortable position on the table supine. The therapist carefully positions their hands in such a way to support the patient's head during distraction. The force is gentle, stable, and controlled.

During traction the therapist may reposition the head to one side, flex, or extend the neck using their hands. A change in head position during traction may affect more positive results in reducing the patient's symptoms.

A mechanical traction device used to treat the cervical spine is comprised of a head halter with over-the-door pulley system. Some patients are allowed to use this system at home after the therapist teaches them how to set the system up, wear the halter, apply the weights correctly, and duration of traction treatment. The patient may be able to use the head halter sitting, reclining, or laying supine.

Lumbar Traction

Manual Lumbar traction involves distracting almost half of the body's weight and therefore requires more of the therapist's strength. After the patient is positioned, the therapist may pull at the ankles, once again using controlled force. Another technique involves draping the patient's legs over the therapist's shoulders. The therapist then steadily pulls with their arms positioned across the patient's thighs. An alternative is a pelvic belt with straps used for distraction.

Mechanical traction may incorporate the use of a motorized split-traction table. The patient is placed in a pelvic harness secured to one end of the table. Some motorized units are computerized enabling the therapist to program the patient's session of therapeutic traction.

Contraindications

When the structural integrity of the spine is compromised, such as in osteoporosis (os-t-o-pour-o-sis), infection, tumor, or cervical rheumatoid arthritis (room-ah-toyed arth-rye-tis), traction is not a treatment option. Physical conditions such as pregnancy, cardiovascular disease, hernia, and in some cases TMJ (temporo-mandibular joint dysfunction or disease, tem-pouro-man-dib-you-lar), exclude patients from spinal traction. In these situations, the forces used in traction (movement) could be potentially dangerous.

Conclusion

Therapeutic spinal traction is not a new concept. Today, the first patient to experience spinal traction would be more than 100 years old! Since then, many studies have been conducted to determine the efficacy of spinal traction. However, these have proved inconclusive.

© SpineUniverse.com. Used with permission.

6

Spine Surgery: Overview

Spine Surgery:
What You Need to Know

Gregory Gilreath, PA-C

The Myth: . . . the only solution
a spine surgeon can offer is surgery.

If you believe the myth you will be interested to learn that out of 100 patients with a back or neck disorder, fewer than 5% require surgery. This means that 95% are treated without surgery.

If a spinal problem falls into the 95% group, the course of treatment may include anti-inflammatory and pain medication, physical therapy, or injection therapy. Certain spinal disorders may require surgical consideration. These include bladder or bowel dysfunction, structural instability, tumor, infection, deformity, progressive neurological deficit, and unrelenting pain that cannot be controlled non-surgically.

In the 5% group, certain spinal disorders arouse more concern. Notably, incapacitating back pain, inability to move an extremity, leg pain, or loss of bladder or bowel control may be signs of progressive and serious neurological dysfunction. In some cases, surgery may be the immediate treatment.

Spine surgery is not the perfect answer or a cure. This type of surgery has its own risks and is quite different from other operations. Not every patient is a candidate for spine surgery. This may relate to the patient's general health. For example, a patient with a

71

cardiac disorder may be at risk during any surgical procedure. If one spine surgery fails, the patient may be advised against additional spine surgery because one failure may lead to another. Smoking and diabetes contributes to the risk for failed spine surgery. Patients who use tobacco are advised to stop at least one month prior to surgery. Nicotine constricts blood vessels slowing circulation, which can inhibit healing. Further, bone does not grow or mend well when nicotine is consumed. People who smoke or use tobacco are apt to have more spine and general health problems.

At one time spine surgery was reserved for younger to middle-aged patients. Today, attitudes have changed, the risks are more controllable, and research has shown that the success rate for elderly patients is as high, or higher, than some younger patients. Sometimes older patients are more motivated to get better. Younger patients may have more underlying problems such as those related to family, employment, stress, and depression. Of course older people share similar problems, but they often have fewer difficulties. During the next 25 years physicians anticipate treating a growing number of elderly patients. Research reveals that the population as a whole is increasing in age.

The Goal of Spine Surgery

The goal of any surgery is to restore the patient's health. Spine surgery is no exception. Spine specialists want to return each patient to his pre- disease or injury functional level quickly. This usually involves relieving the patient's symptoms. In general, the success rates are very good.

Patient Fear When Surgery is Recommended

The thought of spine surgery or any type of operation can frighten some patients. Fear is normal. No one wants to have spine surgery. Fortunately, most spine surgeries are not needed as emergency treatment. Therefore, the patient has the time to learn more about their disorder and the procedure. The patient has the right to decline surgery or obtain a second opinion. These rights are always respected.

When spine surgery is recommended, the spine surgeon discusses the case and proposed surgical plan with the patient's primary care provider (and other specialists, such as the patient's cardiologist). The primary care physician's involvement is important as he is responsible for granting surgical medical clearance.

Patient Surgical Conference

The surgical conference is a meeting between the patient, the surgeon and/or his surgical assistance. The patient is encouraged to bring a family member or friend and to ask questions. Psychologically, a well-informed patient is less anxious about their surgery.

During the meeting, the patient's medical history, test findings, treatments, allergies, and medications are reviewed. The surgeon explains in detail the risks, possible complications, how the surgery is performed, and the patient's expected outcome. The patient is asked to sign an **Informed Consent**. This document outlines in writing the surgical procedure, associated risks and complications, and includes other issues discussed with the surgeon.

Some types of spine surgery can be performed using minimally invasive procedures. These types of procedures appeal to patients because in some cases, the patient may be allowed to go home the same day as their surgery or be released the following day.

Another myth about spine surgery is that a long recuperative period in bed is necessary. This simply is not true. Often the patient is up, out of bed and walking the day after surgery. Even following a complex surgical procedure the patient is up, seated in a chair and walking the next day. Rehabilitation or physical therapy may be started the day after surgery to help the patient become mobile. Many patients are quite independent a short time after spine surgery.

Pre-Operative Tests

A chest x-ray, blood tests, **electrocardiogram** (electro-car-dee-oh-gram), and **urinalysis** (yu-ri-nal-is-sis) are typically included in the patient's pre-operative work-up. If the patient has a co-existing disease such as diabetes, additional tests may be necessary. The primary care physician and/or other treating specialists will be involved to make sure the patient's general health is thoroughly evaluated prior to surgery.

Hospital/Outpatient Pre-Registration

Prior to the surgery day, the hospital or outpatient facility staff will call the patient to schedule an appointment for pre-registration. Pre-registration is a simple process that involves the patient providing information so the treating facility can be paid for services rendered. The type of information needed includes the patient's name, address, social security number, and insurance provider.

Meeting an Anesthesiologist

The patient meets with a member of the anesthesiology department prior to surgery. The anesthesiologist (an-es-thee-z-al-oh-jist) reviews the patient's medical records, discusses the spine surgery and type of sedation to be used during the procedure, and answers the patient's questions.

General anesthesia (general an-es-thee-z-ah) is the usual type of sedation chosen for spine surgery. General anesthesia temporarily affects the central nervous system and helps to keep the patient pain-free and comfortable during surgery.

Pre-Operative Instructions

The surgeon's medical assistant or nurse provides the patient with a written list of instructions to follow before surgery. Instructions include how to prepare the home for post-operative care, planning for the patient's transportation needs, special information about taking current medications, to leave valuables at home, a reminder not to eat or drink anything the evening before surgery, and what time to report to the surgical facility.

Surgery Day

At the surgical facility, the patient checks in and is escorted to a pre-surgical area where the patient is prepared for surgery. Here the patient changes into a hospital gown. The patient's pre-surgical nurse verifies the patient's name, type of surgery to be performed, and reviews their medical history including allergies.

An intravenous line (IV) is started. Different types of necessary medications are injected through the IV into the patient's bloodstream. Light sedating medication may be given to the patient through the IV. Some patients become so relaxed that they do not remember being taken to the operating room.

Operating Room (OR)

The OR is a sterile environment suited with large adjustable overhead lighting, a surgical table, and other equipment. During the operation the anesthesiologist (an-es-thee-z-al-oh-jist) monitors the patient's vital signs—heart rate, blood pressure, and level of sedation. Surgery is a team effort. The surgeon takes the lead and the surgical assistant and nurses support the surgeon and anesthesiologist.

Recovery Room

After surgery the patient is moved into the Recovery Room. Here the patient's vital signs continue to be closely monitored to help minimize post-operative complications. During this time, the surgeon briefly meets with the patient's family. When the patient is stable, he is moved to a hospital room. A patient who had 'same day surgery' is released home only after their post-operative condition is stable and the patient is awake.

Post-Operative Pain and
Patient-Controlled Analgesia (PCA)

Pain following surgery is relative. A patient who has endured pain for years (chronic) may not perceive pain the same way as a patient who has not. Post-operative pain is commonly described as acute pain—it can be severe, but is short-lived.

There are several ways to control post-operative pain; oral medications, intramuscular injections, or Patient-Controlled Analgesia (PCA). PCA puts pain control in the patient's hand. A finger-controlled pumping device feeds pain-relieving medication safely through the patient's IV (intravenous line). The patient simply pushes a button for medication. The pump is programmed with a prescribed amount of medication for a specific time period. It is impossible for the patient to over-medicate.

Walking

Depending on the type of surgery, the patient may be encouraged to walk the next day. Some patients require assistance. Walking and movement increases circulation and enhances healing. Physical therapy may soon be added to help the patient build strength and flexibility. PT usually continues on an outpatient basis after the patient is released from the hospital.

Going Home

Patients are sent home with written instructions and needed prescriptions. The instructions include information about medications, general care at home and hygiene, acceptable post-operative activities, diet, a name and number to call in case of emergency, and surgical follow-up.

Spine Surgery Procedures: A Synopsis
Stewart G. Eidelson, MD

Open Spine Surgery versus Minimally Invasive Spine Surgery

In the past all spine surgeries were 'open' procedures. An open procedure is one that usually requires one or more long incisions, stripping muscle away to reveal bone, greater post-operative pain, and a lengthy recovery period. However, times are quickly changing in the world of spine surgery. Today many spine surgeries are performed through tiny keyhole-type incisions, use specially designed micro-sized instruments, telescope-like endoscopes, video cameras, sophisticated computer-aided imaging systems, and television-type monitors. The trend toward minimally invasive spine surgery is rapidly gaining speed and patients and their surgeons are pleased with the results.

The benefits of a minimally invasive procedure include a few tiny scars instead of one large scar, shorter hospital stay, less post-operative pain, and less recovery time. In many cases, a minimally invasive procedure is just as effective and safe as an 'open' spine surgery.

Today, spinal fusion, deformity correction procedures to treat disorders such as **scoliosis** (sko-lee-oh-sis), and **herniated discs** (her-knee-ate-ed disc) can be treated using minimally invasive technology. Of course there are exceptions—not every patient's spinal disorder is best treated by a minimally invasive procedure.

Discectomy and Microdiscectomy

Microdiscectomy (mycro-dis-eck-toe-me) is the minimally invasive version of the surgical procedure to remove a portion of or an entire intervertebral disc.

Foraminotomy (for-am-not-toe-me)

The **neuroforamen** (nu-row for-a-men) are the nerve passageways through which nerve roots exit the spinal canal. When the size of a neuroforamen is reduced, such as in the case of **spinal stenosis** (spinal sten-oh-sis), a foraminotomy is a procedure used to 'unclog' and reopen the neural (nerve) passageway. A foraminotomy can help to relieve nerve compression, inflammation and pain.

Laminectomy and Laminotomy
(lamb-in-eck-toe-me) and (lamb-in-ah-toe-me)

Both procedures involve the lamina; the thin bony layer covering access to the spinal canal. The difference is 'ectomy' means the complete removal of the lamina, where 'otomy' denotes the partial removal of the bony plate. Removal of a portion of or the entire lamina may be necessary to surgically decompress (remove pressure) from nerve roots. For example, a **herniated disc** (her-knee-ate-ed disc) may compress a nearby nerve root. A laminectomy/otomy may be necessary for the surgeon to gain access to the part of the disc compressing the nerve root. Further, a laminectomy/otomy provides greater access to the spinal canal and other anatomy.

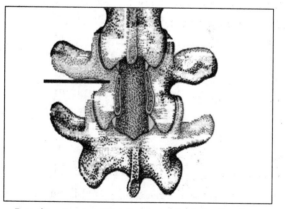

Laminectomy—Total removal of the lamina.

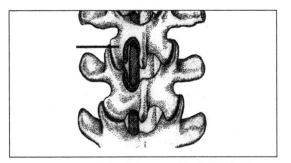

Laminotomy—Partial removal of the lamina.

Spinal Instrumentation and Fusion

Spinal instrumentation is a generic term that refers to surgical procedures that use cages, plates, rods, screws, and other types of implants to stabilize the spine or correct deformity. These devices are made from Titanium alloy or stainless steel and are sometimes called 'hardware'. Conditions that may progress to cause spinal instability include degenerative disc disease, scoliosis (sko-lee-oh-sis), and spondylolisthesis (spon-de-low-lis-thee-sis).

During a spine surgery that includes instrumentation and fusion, bone graft or a bone graft substitute (e.g. biologic material) is placed between the vertebrae and hardware. The bone graft stimulates bone growth that fuses or joins the spine together with the instrumentation into a solid construct.

Some patients must wear a brace following an instrumentation and fusion procedure. The brace helps to support and protect the spine during healing by limiting movement. Periodic x-ray examination of the surgical area is used to monitor the progress of the fusion. Brace use is stopped as soon as the surgeon sees that fusion is successful.

Patients need not fear that an instrumentation and fusion procedure will cause the spine to be stiff and unmovable. Depending on the number of spinal levels fused, some motion may be lost, but this

79

is usually minimal. For example, after a lumbar fusion, the patient is able to bend because most of the motion occurs through the hip joints.

Interbody Cage Fusion

A cage is a small hollow cylindrical device similar in appearance to a birdcage. These devices are called 'interbody cages' because they are placed between two vertebrae in the intervertebral space to replace a disc or to restore disc height. Bone graft (or other biologic material) is packed into and around the cages to stimulate fusion. When the disc space is restored (height added), nerve compression is relieved and symptoms diminish.

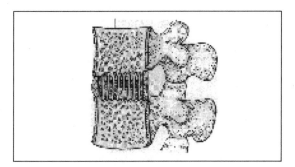

Intervertebral Cage

Anterior (ALIF), Posterior (PLIF), and Transforaminal (TLIF) Lumbar Interbody Fusion

The terms anterior, posterior and transforaminal (trans- foe-ray-men-al) refer to the surgical approach to the spine. Anterior means from the front, posterior from the back or rear, and transforaminal means from the side. Any one of these approaches is used to gain access to a damaged disc. After the disc is surgically removed, an interbody cage and bone graft is placed between the vertebrae to stimulate fusion and stabilize the spine. Depending on the complexity of the case, screws and rods may be implanted to stabilize the spine.

Bone Graft

The different types of bone graft include: autogenous, allograft (al-o-graft), demineralized bone matrix, and bone morphogenetic protein (bone mor-foe-gin-et-ick protein, rh-BMP).

Autogenous Bone Graft is the patient's own bone and is considered the 'gold standard' of bone grafts. During a separate surgical procedure, performed during the primary operation, the surgeon removes pieces of bone from the patient's pelvis or iliac crest (hip area). Autogenous bone provides excellent fusion rates and the risk for the body rejecting its own bone is lower. The disadvantages include the need for an additional surgical incision, increased blood loss, prolonged operating time, and the pain and soreness may last long after the primary surgery has healed.

Allograft Bone Graft is a type of bone graft extender or replacement bone. Allograft (al-o-graft) bone is harvested from deceased individuals who have donated their bone. The disadvantage to allograft bone is that is does not always promote the growth of new bone necessary for a strong and successful fusion.

Demineralized Bone Matrix (DBM) is made of bone growth stimulating proteins demineralized (removed or extracted) from allograft bone. DBM products are used as an 'extender' to the patients own bone (autogenous bone).

Bone Morphogenetic Proteins (BMPs) (bone mor-foe-gin-et-ick proteins) are powerful stimulants that promote bone formation and are used for bone graft replacement. The Food and Drug Administration (FDA) has cleared rhBMP-2 for general used in human spinal fusion.

Bone Growth Stimulators

These devices are used in patients at risk for failed fusion (e.g. diabetics, smokers). There are different types of devices; some are implanted internally and others are worn outside the body. Bone growth stimulators emit electromagnetic waves that stimulate bone tissue to growth and heal.

Image-Guided Spine Surgery

Image-guided procedures combine the technologies of Computer Assisted Surgery (CAS) and Global Positioning Systems (GPS). The spine surgeon can pre-plan a visual map of the patient's surgery and navigate anatomy before and during surgery three-dimensionally in real time.

What are Spinal Instrumentation and Spinal Fusion?

Susan A. Spinasanta

Spinal Instrumentation utilizes surgical procedures to implant Titanium, Titanium-alloy, Stainless Steel, or non-metallic devices into the spine. Instrumentation provides a more permanent solution to spinal instability. Medical implants are specially designed for use in the spine and come in many shapes and sizes. Implants include rods, plates, screws, and interbody cages.

Spinal Fusion is a process that uses bone graft or a biologic material to cause two opposing bony surfaces to grow together. This process is called Arthrodesis. Bone graft can be taken from the patient's pelvis (autogenous bone) during the primary surgical procedure or harvested from other individuals (allograft bone). Bone Morphogenetic Protein (bone mor-foe-gin-et-ick protein, rh-BMP) is new and can be used to stimulate bone growth and spinal fusion.

Instrumentation and Fusion Working Together

Instrumentation maintains spinal stability, which helps to facilitate the fusion process. These procedures help to restore spinal stability, correct deformity (e.g. scoliosis), and bridge or fill space created by the removal of a spinal element (e.g. intervertebral disc).

Both procedures immobilize the involved spinal level(s). This does not necessarily mean the patient is unable to move (e.g. bend over). Many patients state they feel more mobile because their pain has been reduced or eliminated.

An Old Concept Made New

Spinal instrumentation and fusion are not new surgical concepts. Although the first spinal fusion was performed almost 90 years ago, Dr. Paul Harrington developed spinal instrumentation in the late 1950's. During this time, many children stricken with polio developed spinal deformities. In an attempt to treat these children, Dr. Harrington developed the first spinal instrumentation system (Harrington Instrumentation). Rods were secured to the spine at two ends using hooks. The position of the spine was adjusted using a tackling type of device. Through Dr. Harrington's experience, fusion was discovered to be a necessary adjunct to instrumentation. Today, fusion remains an integral part of procedures utilizing instrumentation.

Technology and Technique Progress

During the 1960's instrumentation became more main-stream as doctors, who saw the benefits to patients, found almost 50 ways to modify Harrington's original system. Bone screws and threaded cable were developed. In the 1970's, Dr. Eduardo Luque was using smooth bendable rods and wire to stabilize the spine. Moving into the 1980's instrumentation evolved into a three-dimensional approach to spinal correction. Rods, hooks, and screws were streamlined to meet individual patient needs with less demand on the surgeon to customize implants on the spot.

Today and Tomorrow

Spinal instrumentation systems continue to be redesigned to meet the demands of spine specialists who are true visionaries in this specialized field of surgery. This trend will most certainly continue to provide new and innovative solutions for disorders involving the spine.

Multi Axial Screws Help Make Instrumentation Surgery Easier
Mary Claire Walsh

Introduction

The use of instrumentation—specially designed hooks, rods, and screws—has revolutionized spinal surgery in the last 25 years. As these instrumentation systems continue to develop and progress, millions of patients with a wide variety of serious spinal conditions are finding the help and relief they have been searching for.

Surgeons now have a tool that can help make this type of surgery easier. Medtronic Sofamor Danek's CD HORIZON® M8 Multi Axial Screws are the latest addition to a whole system of instruments designed to stabilize areas of the spine. These specially designed screws facilitate lining up the rods with the pedicle screws. Easier placement means less time spent in surgery for the patient, more successful outcomes, and less recovery time.

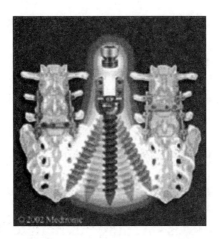

CD HORIZON® M8 Multi Axial Screws
© Medtronic Sofamor Danek. Used with permission.

When Is Instrumentation Used?

Even though most spinal conditions can be treated using non-surgical methods, if the spine becomes too unstable, pain is unresolvable, or the patient experiences neurological dysfunction, surgery may be the best answer.

Instrumentation systems such as hooks, rods, and screws are used to surgically stabilize spinal trauma and deformity. Often, these implants are used together during a procedure—for example, multiaxial screws help with lining up many of the pedicle screws with the rods. Multiaxial screws cut down, to some extent, on the need for rod contouring, they make it easier to engage rods into pedicle screws and they, as stated, cut down on the stress on the bone-screw interface.

There are a variety of spinal conditions that can cause serious spinal instability. These include:

(1) Degenerative spondylolisthesis—a spinal a disorder that causes the forward motion, or slip, of one vertebral body over the one below.

(2) Spinal fracture—breaks in the bones of the spine, such as the vertebrae.

(3) Scoliosis—curvature of the spine.

(4) Kyphosis—a progressive spinal disorder also called humpback or hunchback.

(5) Spinal tumor—cancerous growths on the spine.

If these spinal conditions progress to a point that the spine becomes seriously unstable, instrumentation surgery is performed to add strength and stability, return functionality, and decrease pain.

Screws and Rods—Adding Strength to the Spine

The pedicle is part of the vertebral column that connects the front of the spine to the back of the spine. There is one pedicle on each side of each vertebra. Placing a screw into the pedicle bone of the vertebral body is done to fixate and stabilized the spine. If necessary, pedicle screws can be placed at several levels of the spine; a rod is then used to connect them together, giving the spine considerable extra strength.

How Do These Screws Work?

The CD HORIZON® M8 Multi Axial Screws can be angled 28° in any direction, making it easier for the surgeon to implant hooks, rods or other instrumentation. They also have break-off heads, a feature that helps the surgeon determine when the screws have been successfully secured. Available in medical grade steel and titanium, these "low-profile" screws are designed to fit most body sizes with minimal interference with other parts of the anatomy. In addition, the M8 Multi Axial Screws include a buttress thread design, a single locking mechanism (break off set screws), and top loading mechanism to facilitate rod placement and reduction.

Knowledge is a Powerful Healer

If surgery is necessary, the spine surgeon will discuss with the patient in detail how the procedure will be done. The spine surgeon will determine which instrumentation system is best for the patient's particular condition. While it is not necessary to understand all of the technical aspects of how these instrumentation systems are designed and used, many patients find it helpful and comforting to learn a little about the system used in their procedure. Patients should endeavor to understand as much as they can about their condition and surgery to help them proceed down the road to recovery.

Advanced Nervous System Monitoring during Spine Surgery
Cathleen Zippay, R.EEG/EPT, REDT, CNIM

Neurophysiological monitoring during spine surgery began in the late 1970's. It was found that patients who underwent surgery to correct scoliosis benefited from this special type of neurological testing. Today spine surgeons depend on neurophysiologic intraoperative monitoring to reduce risks during surgery.

The term 'neurophysiologic intraoperative monitoring' refers to the complex process of carefully watching the effects that surgery has on the function of the spinal cord and nerves. This sophisticated form of monitoring is used during high-risk neurosurgical, orthopaedic, vascular and other types of surgeries that may damage the nervous system.

Appropriate monitoring is a team approach between the anesthesiologist, surgeon, monitorist, and interpreting neurophysiologist.

87

Throughout the surgical procedure a certified neurophysiologic technician monitors the function of the patient's nervous system and continuously conveys the results to the surgeon. The purpose of intraoperative monitoring is to prevent injury to vital nerve structures.

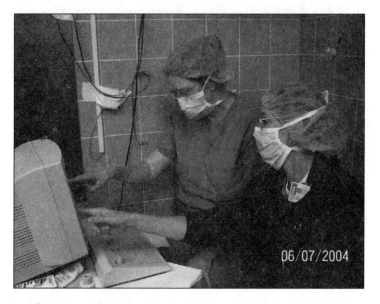

Certified neurophysiologic technicians evaluate a surgical patient.
© Neurometrics. Used with permission.

During surgery, the patient is asleep and is unable to tell the spine surgeon if an arm or leg is numb. Of course there are other symptoms of nerve compromise, but extremity numbness is used here as an example. The sensitive monitoring equipment acts as an early warning system to alert the surgical team to modify the operative procedure to prevent possible irreversible nerve damage.

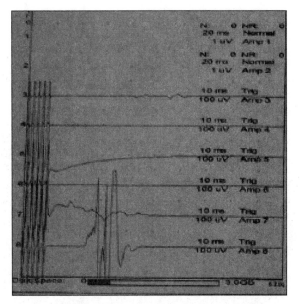

**An example of the 'wave patterns' denoting
nerve function during spine surgery.**

© Neurometrics. Used with permission.

Of course, not all patient anatomy is textbook! Use of this technology gives the surgeon an additional set of eyes and ears to perceive what is going on neurologically during the procedure. For example, neurophysiological intraoperative monitoring can tell the surgeon when the nervous system is not responding well to the patient's position on the surgical table; if nerve root irritation occurs as a pedicle screw is implanted or during rod insertion to correct abnormal curvature of the spine; or, a bone graft is too large for the space between two intervertebral bodies.

Bottom line—It is all about reducing the patient's risk for nerve impairment during surgery and increasing the opportunity for a good outcome.

7

Cervical Spine Surgery and Devices

The Cervical Spine: Degenerative Disorders and Treatment

Steven R. Garfin, MD
Christopher M. Bono, MD

Introduction

At one time or another, most people have experienced neck pain. In the vast majority of cases, this is a benign, self-limited complaint. Symptoms are commonly described as a soreness or stiffness of the neck, which may or may not be associated with a minor injury. Patients often attribute this to a 'cold wind' or 'sleeping wrong' that may or may not be a factor. Most commonly, degenerative disorders of the spine are responsible. Degenerative 'disease' is the change associated with spinal wear and tear or age. Through among the most frequent causes of neck pain, it is sometimes the most difficult to treat.

Other possible disorders that can cause neck pain are **rheumatoid arthritis** (room-ah-toyed arth-rye-tis), infection, or cancer. It is rare that such conditions cause only neck pain, as they are usually associated with other warning signs such as profound or unintentional weight loss, fevers, or pain in other joints such as the hips or knees.

The focus of this chapter is a discussion of degenerative

disorders of the cervical spine. These affect adult patients of any age, with a tendency for particular disorders to affect certain age groups.

Cervical disc **herniations** (her-knee-ate-shuns) are more characteristic in the young (less than 40-years old), while cervical **spondylosis** (spon-dee-low-sis) and **stenosis** (sten-oh-sis) are typically found in older patients. Treatments vary from observation, medications, and therapy to injections or operative intervention.

Definition: Degenerative Disease

As a patient, the first question is obvious. *What is degenerative disease of the spine?* In all honestly, the academic leaders of the spine world are currently pondering this same question. What we mean is that spine doctors can recognize and treat degenerative disorders of the spine but are often unclear how the disorder actually arises except to attribute it to age. To date, most theories about how the spine degenerates remain that—theories. Although these theories are often well thought out and reasonable, it is exceedingly difficult to prove them, as they are the best explanation we have to explain degenerative disease of the spine at this time.

Degenerative disease of the spine refers to a break down of the normal architecture of the various components of the cervical spine. Normally, the neck is very flexible. As you may demonstrate on yourself, the neck allows the head to rotate from side-to-side nearly 180 degrees, to flex forward to touch your chin to your chest, and extend backward to almost touch the back of the head to your upper back, as well as bend your head toward your shoulder (and all ranges in between these basic motions). These motions are afforded by the various joints of the cervical spine.

There are seven cervical bones in the spine. Known as vertebrae (ver-ta-bray, plural of vertebra), they can be likened to the cars of a passenger train. The cars of the train, by themselves, are stiff with no ability to bend. Each car (vertebrae) is joined to its neighbor by a joint. The joint allows motion between the cars. As in the spine, joining a number of cars together can allow overall motion. The more joints and vertebrae, the more motion is allowed. In contrast to the joints of the car, the cervical vertebrae are connected by three joints. This gives the spine more stability, while still allowing motion. The extremes of motion must be limited because of the fragile 'freight' that the vertebrae hold—the spinal cord. Like the people in the cars of the train, the spinal cord is located in the center of the vertebrae.

At this point, clarification of terms is important. Spine refers to the bony parts. These are the vertebrae that were described above. Spinal cord is the nerve elements that travel within the spine from the brain down to the rest of the body. The spinal cord transmits signals (bioelectrical and biochemical) that control all the functions (muscles and sensations) below that level. The function of the spine is to protect the spinal cord from injury during motion and activity.

Joints are comprised of two opposing surfaces of bone. Some joints are covered with smooth, glistening cartilage (car-til-ledge). The slippery properties of cartilage make the two surfaces move easily in relation to each other. The **facet joints** (fah-set joint) of the cervical spine have these properties.

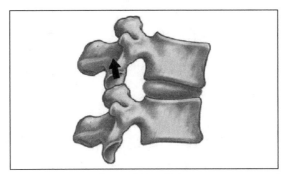

Upper Facet Joint
© SpineUniverse.com. Used with permission.

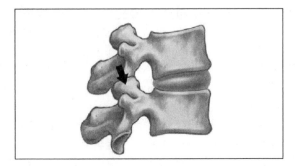

Lower Facet Joint
© SpineUniverse.com. Used with permission.

In contrast, the main joint between two cervical vertebrae is made up by a large spongy mass, the intervertebral disc. This disc sits between the two broad flat surfaces of the vertebral bodies. This disc is made up of specialized materials that act as soft 'glue' between the bones, while still allowing them to move. The disc is extremely important to spinal stability. However, it is a frequent site of degeneration or breakdown.

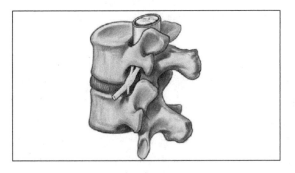

Vertebral Segment
© SpineUniverse.com. Used with permission.

In another way, the disc can be considered as a pillow between two bones. The pillows can softly resist the downward forces placed on the vertebrae from the weight and movement of the head. A good pillow is thick and soft and functions best. It allows some movement between the vertebrae. Because the pillow is well fixed to both bones, it resists the tendency of the bones to become misaligned. With time and use the pillow can become flattened.

In this state the disc no longer provides adequate cushioning between the vertebrae. The bones then come closer and closer together. Because the disc is no longer sustaining the forces that it usually does, the other joints of the spine are forced to take on these extra loads. The two smaller sliding joints (**facet joints**, fah-set) have greater demands placed on them. Since they were designed to sustain only a small portion of the forces of the spine, the previously glistening, healthy cartilage starts to breakdown. As the cartilage degenerates, the underlying bone becomes exposed and an inflammatory reaction begins. This causes irritation of the joint, which can lead to pain. This sets up a vicious cycle of events. The more the facet joints become degenerated, the less they are able to tolerate the increased demands. Thus, greater demands will then be placed on the intervertebral disc, causing it to further degenerate (or breakdown) as well. The changes in the intervertebral disc and facet joints are not reversible at this time.

Common Disorders

An important feature of disc degeneration is the reaction that the bone undergoes. Because the normal relationships of the bones are lost, there is a condition of instability. This refers to one vertebra moving in an abnormal manner in relation to the next vertebra. To attempt to stabilize this excess motion, bone grows outward. These outward growths are called **osteophytes** (os-t-o-fights). Osteophytes can be found near the disc spaces and around the facet joints. Osteophytes take up space. If they grow in areas where nerves or the spinal cord are nearby, they can impinge or compress these structures. This can cause pain, numbness, tingling, or weakness to varying degrees. If significant enough to cause nerve dysfunction, it is known as cervical stenosis (sten-oh-sis).

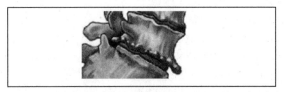

Osteophyte formation near the disc and joint.
© SpineUniverse.com. Used with permission.

Cervical Disc Herniation

Disc degeneration can sometimes follow a slightly difference course. In the process of sustaining increased mechanical loads, the outer aspect of the disc, known as the **annulus** (an-you-lus), can become stressed. This outer ring normally keeps the soft, gel-like center of the disc contained. The gel center, known as the **nucleus** (new-klee-us) can be ejected from the disc through an annular tear. This is called a disc herniation. If the disc herniates in the direction of the spinal cord or nerve root, it can cause neurologic compromise. Disc herniations in the cervical spine can be serious. If significant enough, they can cause **paralysis** (pa-ral-eh-sis) of both the upper and lower extremities, though this is extremely rare.

In most cases, a patient complains of neck pain associated with **radiating** (ray-dee-ating) pain to one arm. This is caused by compression of a nerve root, rather than the spinal cord itself. With time some herniated discs resolve or shrink by themselves. Sometimes, disc herniations can persist, causing prolonged symptoms and neurologic problems, which may lead to surgical considerations.

Cervical Spondylosis

This rather elaborate sounding word is really nothing more than a description of what happens to the vast majority of our cervical spines as we get older. The term **spondylosis** (spon-dee-low-sis) refers to the bony overgrowths associated with aging of the spine. Though it is hypothesized, as discussed, that **osteophytes** (os-t-o-fights) form because of micro-instability and disc degeneration, this is not certain. It is known that a high percentage of patients without any neck pain or other symptoms have spondylosis of the spine. In some people however, spondylosis may be associated with neck pain. Spondylosis is likely the end result of disc degeneration that has been present for a very long time.

Differential Diagnosis

What else can be causing my neck pain?

Diagnosing degenerative disorders of the spine starts with a good history and physical examination. Typically, patients have neck pain. This is the most common complaint. Unfortunately, neck pain is a common complaint in the vast majority of people who have nothing more than a stiff neck. It is important to differentiate neck pain related to degenerative spinal disorders from other more serious ailments.

Muscle **strains** can cause mild pain. This can vary from the occasional 'stiff neck' (from keeping your neck in one position too long such as during sleep) to neck soreness associated with a low-speed motor vehicle collision (**whiplash**). The pain and tenderness is not deep and is usually limited to the surrounding muscles around the neck. Often, one side is more symptomatic that the other. Muscles strains are differentiated from degenerative disorders by their self-limited course. Muscle strains usually resolve, or at least dramatically improve, within a couple of day to weeks. Pain that continues for more than three weeks without improving may not be a muscle strain and other diagnoses should be considered.

Patients with **rheumatoid arthritis** (room-ah-toyed arth-rye-tis) can have neck pain. It is important to recognize this. Any patient with rheumatoid arthritis should have neck x-rays taken. These patients can develop instability in the upper cervical spine that can endanger the spinal cord. This is easily recognized on plain x-rays.

Neck pain can be a presenting symptom of meningitis (men-in-ji-tis), an infection of the brain and spinal cord linings. Meningitis can have many causes and may be contagious. Although neck pain is probably the most common symptom, it is important to recognize the other signs. Patients often are extremely sensitive to light, irritable, have high fevers, and actually tolerate very little movement of the neck. Though it is rare, this diagnosis is very serious and should prompt an individual to seek urgent medical care. Other types of infections can also occur in the neck. Infection can occur in the bone or intervertebral disc. This is more common in older patients who may have a weak immune system. Again, as with meningitis a history of fever could be important, but there is not hypersensitivity to bright light.

Tumors can also cause neck pain. One way to clinically differentiate tumor from degenerative disorders is the presence of generalized or constitutional symptoms. Unintentional weight loss, feeling of extreme lethargy, persistent low grade fevers, and night sweats are typical constitutional symptoms. A history of cancer elsewhere is also a clue, as the majority of neck tumors are metastases (or spread, ma-tax-ta-sees) from a cancer in the lung, prostate, kidney or breast.

Typical Cases

Cervical Stenosis

As discussed above, cervical stenosis means, literally, tightening or narrowing of the canal around the spinal cord. Of the degenerative disorders discussed in this chapter, it is potentially the most serious. If the cervical stenosis (sten-oh-sis) is profound enough, it can cause dysfunction of the spinal cord known as myelopathy (my-il-lop-ah-thee). The typical person who has cervical stenosis and myelopathy may be in his or her fifties or sixties. The patient often has complained of neck pain for many years. In some cases, the pain can actually be mild. Therapy may have been prescribed, in addition to medications for the pain. The other features of this disorder will be demonstrated in an illustrative case.

Presentation

Mrs. S is a 61-year old woman with a long-term complaint of neck pain. In the past, her pain has been amply controlled with ibuprofen (Motrin™) and some home exercises. Occasionally she wears a soft cervical collar to calm her neck spasms. She is an avid knitter and has made several sweaters and scarves for her grandchildren recently. In the past two months however, she finds that her fingers are becoming clumsy and she had to take frequent breaks. In addition, Mrs. S is finding that she is not as agile buttoning her blouses in the morning. She is not complaining of any pain in the arms or legs. Interestingly, her legs are a bit wobbly, but she attributes that to some arthritis that has set in over the years. Mrs. S has had no problems urinating on her own and no change in her bowel habits or control.

Examination

At the doctor's office she is given a full examination. She has a somewhat decreased range of motion of the neck with some pain at the extremes of the movements. She walks with an abnormal gait, which can be described as 'wide-based'. In looking at her feet during ambulation, her feet are more spread apart than normal and she stumbles a bit with some steps. Her reflexes in her arms and legs are very jumpy. This is termed **hyperreflexia** (hi-per-ref-flex-e-ah). She does not have any noticeable weakness in the arms or legs. Because of these findings, the doctor gets some x-rays in the office.

Diagnostic Tests

The plain x-rays show a degenerative spine. As discussed above, this can be better termed as **spondylosis** (spon-dee-low-sis). She

99

has **osteophytes** (os-t-o-fights) in the front and back of the spine, which might be protruding into the spinal canal. From the x-ray, there does not appear to be any masses or lesions that would suggest a tumor or infection. Mrs. S's doctor knows that these bony changes are very common at her age. Also, he understands that the plain x-ray is not a very good way of assessing the spinal cord or the space around it.

Mrs. S is sent for an **MRI** scan of her neck. This test entails her lying down for about 45-minutes in a long tube. The long tube has a very large magnet in it. This is what is responsible for the magnet part of magnetic resonance imaging (MRI). Because different tissues in the body respond to magnetic fields in different way, they have characteristic appearances on MR images.

Mrs. S's MRI showed severe narrowing of her spinal canal. Most of this narrowing is coming from degenerated discs that are protruding into the spinal canal. These discs appear hard and have bony osteophytes above and below them, making the compression even less forgiving.

Specialist Consultation

After getting the MRI report, Mrs. S's doctor sends her to a spine surgeon. She explains to the patient that her condition is called cervical stenosis. Because her stenosis or tightening is severe, the nerves in the spinal cord cannot function normally. The compression of the spinal cord is causing her to fumble with her knitting needles and blouse buttons, as well as giving her 'wobbly' legs. This surprises Mrs. S the most, as she was sure that she had knee arthritis that was causing her leg symptoms. The spine surgeon explained that the nerves that go to both the arms and legs pass through the neck within the spinal cord. Thus, compression at the neck can causes symptoms in the arms and legs.

Asking what can be done about her condition, the spine surgeon explains that it is likely that her finger and leg fumbling can get worse. In fact, the tightening around the spinal cord can get to the point that she may lose control of her bladder and bowel. In the best case scenario her symptoms will stay the same for the rest of her life, which can be expected in a low percentage of patients.

The treatment options given to Mrs. S are that she can be treated non-operatively or by surgery. The surgeon explains what comprises non-operative treatment. It includes non-steroidal medications (such as Motrin™, Naprosyn™), physical therapy for the neck muscles, cervical collar use, and traction. Of the options, Mrs. S was most concerned about traction, as she would have to be lying down for a portion of the day while the weights were attached to her chin and head.

Mrs. S was informed of the surgical options. Because of the extent of her disease, the surgeon explained that the best method of relieving the pressure on the spinal cord was to remove the bone from the front of the neck and off the spinal cord. This is known as a **corpectomy** (core-peck-toe-me).

A corpectomy would entail an incision in the front of the neck through which the surgeon can remove the parts of the vertebral bodies that are compressing the spinal cord. In place of the vertebral bodies, a large piece of bone from her own pelvis, or a cadaver donor (**allograft**, al-o-graft) would be inserted. This bone would be expected to heal in place. This is known as a fusion. The likelihood of catching any disease from the cadaver bone is extremely low and is in fact much lower than contracting any disease from a blood transfusion. The more significant risks were from the surgery itself, she was told.

The possible complications include damage to the large arteries that supply blood to the brain and to the spinal cord. Spinal cord damage may cause Mrs. S to be completely paralyzed from the neck down. She was informed that these are the most serious complications. Other complications such as infection is possible, but are more easily treated. Damage to the nerves that supply the vocal cords is also a potential complication. Mrs. S was made aware of this possibility and that she could have hoarseness permanently after the operation. After hearing the options, Mrs. S asks the spine surgeon a few key questions.

First, *if she has damage to her spinal cord already, what are the chances of her symptoms getting better with surgery?*

Because she is still highly functional, she has a good chance of resolving some symptoms, though perhaps not all of her neurologic symptoms. Her neck pain, though not the focus of surgery, may or may not get better. If the surgery is a complete success, she will be able to return to her previous activities with a greatly decreased chance of her spinal cord being further compressed. In essence, the surgery is mostly to keep her from progressively getting worse and/or prevent a catastrophic event like a spinal cord injury could result with a very minor injury such as a slip and fall.

What will happen to her if she doesn't choose surgery?

From the studies available, it is probable that Mrs. S's cervical stenosis will worsen with time. Although it is possible that she could live the rest of her life without any advancement of her problems, it is unlikely. Furthermore, it is even more unlikely for her neurologic symptoms to significantly improve.

What happens if the piece of bone doesn't heal in place?

This is a rather common complication occurring in about 15 to 20 percent of patients undergoing this procedure. In the event that the bone doesn't fuse in the front, a second surgery to fuse the back of the vertebrae is performed. This is done through an incision along the back of the neck.

Outcome

Weighing the options and contemplating the possible complications of both operative and non-operative treatment, Mrs. S decides to proceed with surgery. Thankfully, the surgery was without complication. After surgery, she remained in the hospital for three days. Her neck was very sore but strong pain medication helped to manage the pain. She was instructed to keep a hard cervical collar (**brace**) on at all times for six weeks. She was able to get out of bed the day after surgery and started to eat a full diet as tolerated. After she was discharged, she followed up with her surgeon in the office. The wound healed well. After six weeks she did not use the cervical collar any more. The bone graft showed good signs of healing to her bone on the x-rays. After three months she felt that her fingers were working better and she no longer felt wobbly in the legs. She returned to knitting producing a blue baby bonnet for her newborn grandson.

Cervical Herniated Disc

Just as in the lumbar spine, cervical spine discs can herniate and cause pain, numbness, tingling or even spinal cord compression. Typically patients complain of neck pain associated with pain radiating into one arm. This is termed **radiculopathy** (rah-dick-u-lop-ah-thee). Patients who have herniated cervical discs are younger and often more active than those with cervical stenosis. The disc herniation may be associated with a particular incident, such as a sudden jerking movement or positioning of the neck. Both non-operative and surgical treatment methods can be effective in relieving symptoms.

Presentation

Mr. D is a 35-year old man who has a recent onset of neck and right arm pain. He has had neck pain for about six months, while the arm pain is more recent. Mr. D also describes some numbness is the right hand, which he attributes to carpal tunnel syndrome. Though he had never been diagnosed with carpal tunnel syndrome, he seemed to have very similar symptoms as a good friend of his who was recently diagnosed with this disorder.

He is very active, lifts weights and runs about two miles daily before working as an accountant. He does not have any other symptoms. He has no other significant medical problems. Mr. D has no bladder or bowel complaints. He has never sought medical care for his neck pain, which to him is more significant than his arm pain. The arm pain comes and goes, but is tolerable. The neck pain, on occasion prevents him from going to work. Usually one day off with a brief course of aspirin works to relieve the pain. Running does not seem to aggravate it and his weight lifting exercises seems to temporarily decrease the pain. He seeks medical attention because he feels the onset of arm pain may be related to his neck.

Examination

His primary care doctor examines Mr. D. He has near full range of motion of the neck with some mild tenderness along the muscles of the back of the neck. In **palpating** (pal-pay-ting, feeling) the back of the neck, it seems that he has some tenderness in the midline. The doctor believes this to be in the area of the C5-6 vertebrae. The shoulders, elbows and wrists also have good range of motion and do not appear to have pain associated with their movement.

The neurologic examination demonstrates that Mr. D has some decreased sensitivity of his thumb and along the outer forearm. He does not exhibit any weakness or abnormal reflexes. The remainder of his examination is normal. Because of the numbness and the suggestion of carpal tunnel syndrome by the patient, the doctor orders an **EMG** (**electromyography** test, elec-tro-mypah-gra-fee) of his upper extremities.

Diagnostic Tests

The EMG demonstrated what is known as cervical **radiculopathy** (rah-dick-u-lop-ah-thee). In brief, the EMG is a test of nerve function in the arms and hands. Based on the distribution of nerve abnormalities, the electromyographer can determine if nerves are being compressed in the hand, elbow, shoulder or cervical spine. Because nerves are continuous structures, they can also be compressed in more than one location. Mr. D's EMG showed no evidence of nerve compression within the arm itself, but rather that the nerves were compressed in the spine. This is known as radiculopathy.

With the EMG results, the primary care doctor is now concerned about a correlation between Mr. D's arm and neck symptoms. He then orders x-rays of the neck and an MRI of the cervical spine (doctors love to exchange medical words with lay terms—thus neck means the same as cervical spine). Believing that Mr. D may have significant findings on the MRI, he sends his patient to see a spine surgeon.

Specialist Consultation

The spine surgeon examines the patient and agrees with the primary care doctor's assessment. There is a definite numbness along the thumb and outer aspect of the right forearm. This is the area to which a particular nerve, C6 supplies sensation. Thus he would expect to find compression of this nerve on the MRI. Looking over the EMG results, the electromyographer found that C6 nerve root function was altered on the right side compared to the left; an indication that the nerve is being compressed. The plain x-rays did not show any abnormalities and were deemed normal. The MRI however was a bit more interesting. The radiologist detected a small herniation of one of the cervical intervertebral discs. The disc herniated on the right side was compressing the C6 nerve root. There was no compression of the spinal cord and there did not appear to be any other disc herniations.

The spine surgeon discussed the diagnosis with Mr. D. He stated that what he had was a cervical disc **herniation** (her-knee-aye-shun) and this was causing his arm numbness. It has probably been developing over a period of time and likely explains his six months of neck pain. It is understandable that the disc may have started to degenerate over time and that finally the nucleus (new-klee-us) of the disc popped out. This was the time of the onset of arm pain.

Mr. D was a bit confused at this time. *Why was the other doctor calling his problem a radiculopathy when he really had a herniated disc?* The surgeon explained that in actuality the herniated cervical disc is causing the **radiculopathy**. In other words, the term radiculopathy indicates that the nerve is being pinched. This usually occurs because of a herniated disc but can happen in other disorders too.

Mr. D is now concerned about what to do about his condition. He tells the spine surgeon that he can live with the pain and numbness in the arm and that he knows what to do for his neck ache when it flares up. Basically, the pain is tolerable. The surgeon reassures Mr. D that if he can tolerate the pain, he can continue his regular activities. If he so desired, he could start a course of **physical therapy** to strengthen his neck muscles and increase their flexibility, but he is probably doing a good job of it in the gym on his own. The surgeon does inform him that good non-steroidal anti-inflammatory medications are available over the counter, though therapeutic doses may vary. Additionally, there are many other medications that can be prescribed.

Mr. D was given another non-surgical option called an **epidural** (ep-e-do-ral) steroid injection. This entails an injection into the space around the spinal cord and nerve roots in the neck. The injection can be directed to the particular nerve root that is compressed by a herniated disc. It is effective in about 60% of cases and, as the surgeon explained it is not an unreasonable alternative to surgery.

The surgeon does inform Mr. D of an operation to relieve nerve compression called a cervical **discectomy** (dis-eck-toe-me) and fusion. Similar to Mrs. S's operation, it involves an incision in the front part of the neck to gain access to the intervertebral disc. The disc is then removed and a piece of bone graft is placed in between the two bones (vertebrae). This causes the bones to fuse together into one large bone. The same risks and complications are explained to Mr. D, which include paralysis, infection, bleeding, and failed bone healing. Mr. D appeared quite frightened of the procedure and immediately rejected the idea of it.

After further contemplation, Mr. D asked what about the benefits of this type of surgery. The surgeon told Mr. D that if the herniation were located more laterally (to the side) another option would be an operation through the back of his neck. This would be a **laminotomy** (lamb-in-ah-toe-me, removing a small part of the bony lamina) to gain access to the spinal nerve, moving it and taking out only the herniated component of the disc.

The surgeon explained to Mr. D that the operation, if completely successful, would be most effective in relieving the arm pain and numbness. The relief of his neck pain would be more variable, but he would have a good chance of relieving that as well. The danger of not having the operation is minimal.

In other words, *what would happen if the disc herniation got worse and compressed the nerve even more?* The surgeon informed Mr. D that if his weakness got worse and he started to have other symptoms such as wobbly legs and problems with finger coordination, that he should return to the office soon. These symptoms could be an indication that the disc has protruded farther into the spinal canal and may be compressing the nerves and possibly the spinal cord. If this occurred, the surgeon recommends surgery. However, he assured Mr. D this rarely occurs.

If the arm and neck pain is tolerable and the nerve function stays the same or improves, there is no need for surgery. This is the option Mr. D chooses. Since seeing the spine surgeon, he has been taking his medication when he experiences pain. His numbness actually improved over the next couple of months. He has remained active in his jogging and weightlifting, although the latter may not be mechanically 'friendly' to his spine as aerobic exercise.

Cervical Spondylosis

Cervical spondylosis (sir-ve-kal spon-dee-low-sis) can be thought of as 'grey hair' of the spine. This means that if you live long enough (and that may only mean 40- to 50-years of age in some populations) x-rays of your spine will eventually show signs of cervical spondylosis.

As described above, the term refers to **osteophytes** (os-t-o-fights) or **bony overgrowths** that protrude from the vertebral bodies as well as narrowing occurring across the disc spaces as the disc degenerates. Though osteophytes can compress the spinal cord (like Mrs. S) or a spinal nerve root (like Mr. D), the vast majority of these bony overgrowths do not cause any nerve problems. However, they are a sign that the disc between the vertebrae and facets has become degenerative.

Degenerative discs can cause pain. Unfortunately, the mechanism of pain is not well understood. Pain is thought to be transmitted by tiny nerve endings that innervate the back part of the disc and facet joints. Degeneration can cause pain from the disc, facet joint, or both concomitantly. Diagnostic efforts are aimed at determining which of these structures generates pain. Therapy is directed at relieving the stress placed on these areas.

Presentation

Mrs. P is a 42-year old woman who was involved in a motor vehicle accident 10 years ago. Since then, her neck has never felt 'right'. She has frequent neck spasms that cause her to miss many days of work as an assembly line worker. Mrs. P states her neck pain frequently radiates to the base of her head and down into her shoulder blades. She has no arm or leg pain, bladder or bowel complaints, and no problems hand or feet coordination.

Mrs. P has taken many medications over the past 10 years. During the first couple of years ibuprofen was working adequately. About seven years ago, an emergency room doctor gave her a shot of Demerol™, which she felt disagreed with her but, did temporarily relieve her pain. Two weeks later the pain returned. Her primary care doctor began to prescribe a mild narcotic Vicodin™ about three years ago. She takes this on occasion but, she does not like the 'spacey' feeling it causes. She has had two courses of physical therapy in the past. In describing the therapy she states she was given exercises concentrating on extending her neck. She felt this made her pain worse despite the therapist's reassurance that this would help relieve the pressure across her intervertebral discs. Mrs. P refuses to go back to physical therapy.

Her primary care doctor also instructed Mrs. P to use a home traction set up. The traction device is attached to the top of a door and Mrs. P uses traction in an upright seated position. The device consists of a chin-head strap connected to a rope that runs over a pulley. The other end of the rope is connected to light weights (five to 10 pounds) which deliver an upward force along Mrs. P's neck. When she is in traction, she experiences some relief but, it is short lived. The pain usually returns 30-minutes after she has stopped traction. Mrs. P also uses a soft cervical collar when she has extreme neck spasms. Again the relief is temporary. She returns to her primary care doctor for a regular visit and to discuss the options for her excruciating neck pain.

Examination

Mrs. P's primary care doctor performs a careful neurologic exam that shows no abnormal nerve function. Her neck is stiff with a markedly decreased range of motion. She notices that when the doctor was testing extension (head to the back) the pain worsened.

Diagnostic Tests

Over the years, Mrs. P has had numerous x-rays of the spine. Her latest x-ray showed degenerative changes with multiple **osteophytes** (os-t-o-fights) growing from the front and back of the C5 and C6 vertebral bodies. An MRI of her neck, taken one year ago showed no nerve or spinal cord compression but, shortening of the intervertebral disc height. This suggests that the disc has become dried and degenerated and that it is not functioning normally.

More importantly, there appears to be degeneration of the **facet joints** (fah-set joints) as well at the C5 and C6 levels. After having treated Mrs. P's painful neck for many years to no avail, her doctor has decided to seek a specialist consultation from a pain management doctor.

Specialist Consultation

The pain management doctor reviews Mrs. P's records, chart, x-rays and MRI. His examination demonstrates that her pain is worse with extension of the neck. He tells her that she has what appears to be degenerative cervical **spondylosis** (sir-ve-kal spon-dee-low-sis) at the C5-6 level. Because her neck pain is worse with extension, the doctor believes that Mrs. P has pain associated with facet arthritis (fah-set arth-rye-tis). He suggests that she undergo a series of injections into the facet joints to determine if this decreases her pain. The injections would be Lidocaine™ (a numbing medicine) and corticosteroids (anti-inflammatory medicine). She agrees with this plan.

The injections into the facet joint at C5-6 gave Mrs. P substantial relief. She has seen the pain doctor two more times over the past 10 months since her initial visit. Each time the facet injection helps to relieve her pain dramatically to the point where she can skip taking her pain medicines some days. Unfortunately, the effects have only lasted about three months after each injection.

The pain doctor is confident that her 'pain generator' is the facet joint at C5-6 (cervical spine). He explains to Mrs. P that if the pain continues she might be interested in surgery to fuse the two vertebrae together. This would eliminate motion at the painful joint and hopefully relieve her pain. The doctor explains that the procedure has approximately a 70% success rate in providing long lasting pain relief. He states that he does not perform the surgery and that Mrs. P would need a referral to a spine surgeon. Mrs. P thinks about her options carefully. Although her pain continues, she is not willing to undergo surgery yet. Since the injections provide temporary relief she feels that she has been able, to a degree, resume her regular activities. Since this is the first time in 10 years that she has had improvement in her symptoms, she would like to postpone surgery for as long as possible. The doctor agreed with her decision. Surgery on the neck for neck pain is not nearly as reliable in relieving pain as is surgery on the neck to decrease arm pain.

Conclusion

Degenerative disorders of the spine continue to be a significant cause of neck pain in today. The understanding of these problems continues to grow. With that—patient understanding should follow suit. Affected patients should be aware of the possible treatment modalities including medication, therapy, bracing, selective injections, and surgery. The best patient is one that is informed who understands the natural progression of these disorders as well as the benefits, risks and complications of treatment.

For more information about the cervical spine, disorders, non-surgical and surgical treatments, go to: *www.spineuniverse.com*

Aesculap® CCR:
Caspar Cervical Retractor System
Aesculap, Inc.

Retractors have been used by surgeons for years. The benefits of retractor use include: ensures stable access to the surgical site, provides good visibility, and enables the surgeon to perform the operation without hand retraction.

Pictured on page 112 is the Caspar Cervical Retractor that is part of a system of retracting instruments that includes a separate retractor for use during lumbar spine surgery.

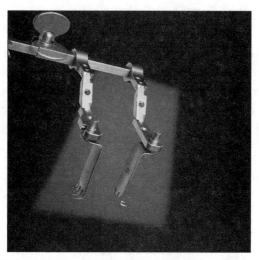

Caspar Cervical Retractor surgical instrument.

© Aesculap®. Used with permission.

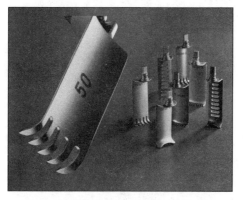

**Range of blade lengths and widths
to suit the surgeon's needs.**

© Aesculap®. Used with permission.

Blackstone™ 3° Anterior Cervical Plate System

Blackstone Medical, Inc.

Degenerative disc disease, spinal stenosis, and trauma can cause the cervical spine (neck) to become unstable. The 3° Anterior Cervical Plate System (Blackstone™ Medical Inc.) is used to stabilize C2-C7. The 3° plate has one of the lowest plate profiles in the market. This means the plate lies very flat against the spine. The plate, screws, and locking plates are made from titanium alloy.

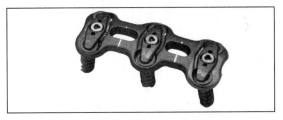

3° Anterior Cervical Plate System.

© Blackstone™ Medical Inc. Used with permission.

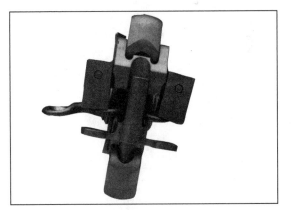

Surgeon bends the 3° Anterior Cervical Plate to fit the contour of the patient's cervical spine.

© Blackstone™ Medical Inc. Used with permission.

113

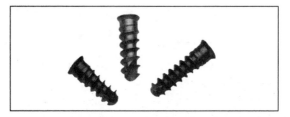

Screws are color-coded and come in many lengths.

© Blackstone™ Medical Inc. Used with permission.

The plate, screws and top locking plates "construct" a stable cervical spine. Two types of locking plates (see below) allow the surgeon to choose the degree of constraint built into the construct. The terms *constrained, unconstrained* or *semi-constrained* may be used to denote the degree of screw movement allowed.

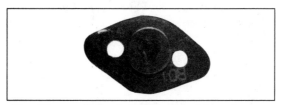

The "Bronze" Top Locking plate is used when constructing a constrained or unconstrained plate construct.

© Blackstone™ Medical Inc. Used with permission.

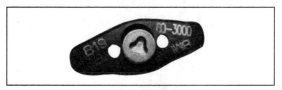

The "Blue" Top Locking Plate is used when constructing a semi-constrained plate construct.

© Blackstone™ Medical Inc. Used with permission.

Three post-operative x-rays demonstrate the appearance of the 3° Anterior Cervical Plate after surgery. In all three cases, the patients' symptoms were alleviated and each patient is doing well.

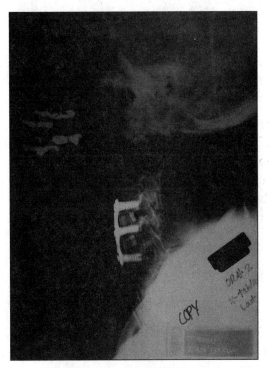

Figure A. Lateral (side) view
Clinical Case. Courtesy Jeffrey Gross, M.D.
Neurological Surgery Community
Orthopedic Medical Group, Mission Viejo, CA

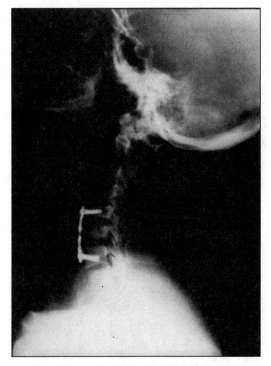

Figure B. Lateral (side) view
Clinical Case. Courtesy Jeffrey Gross, M.D.
Neurological Surgery Community
Orthopedic Medical Group, Mission Viejo, CA

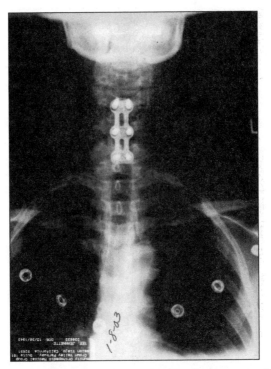

Figure C. AP view; front (anterior) to back (posterior)
Clinical Case. Courtesy Jeffrey Gross, M.D.
Neurological Surgery Community
Orthopedic Medical Group, Mission Viejo, CA

The Cyclone® Anterior Cervical Plate
Encore Medical Corporation

The Cyclone® Anterior Cervical Plate is made by Encore Medical, L.P. The product is a low profile design, which means it lies more flat against the cervical spine. The instruments the surgeon uses and the bone screws are color-coded for quick and easy identification. This versatile system offers different sized plates and bone screws.

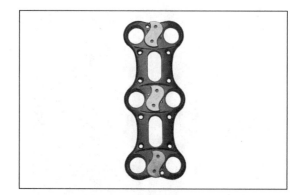

This Cyclone® Plate would be used in a two-level neck fusion.
Encore Medical, L.P. Used with permission.

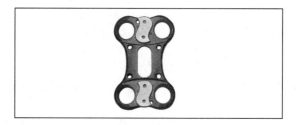

This Cyclone® Plate would be used in a single-level neck fusion.
Encore Medical, L.P. Used with permission.

EBI® VueLock® Anterior Cervical Plate System
EBI

The VueLock® cervical plate system designed by EBI is implanted to stabilize the neck. The plates are low profile, which means the device lays flatter against spinal structures and minimizes irritation to soft tissues (Fig. 1 and 2). The cervical plates are pre-contoured to suit the patient's individual anatomy.

118

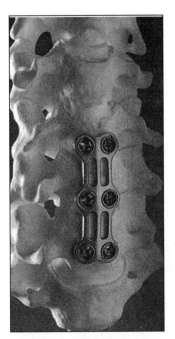

Figure 1. The VueLock® is a low profile cervical plate system.

© EBI. Used with permission.

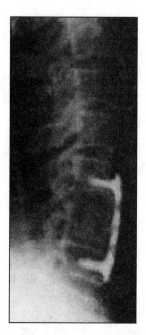

**Figure 2. A lateral post-operative view
of an implanted VueLock® cervical plate.**

© EBI. Used with permission.

The components of the VueLock® plate system are made from titanium alloy, which is strong and compatible to x-ray and other types of imaging studies (e.g. CT Scan).

The screw and locking mechanism is simple and efficient. *Variable angle screw placement* gives the spine surgeon flexibility to precisely position the screw. This is demonstrated in Figures 3 and 4 below. Notice how flat the screw head locks against the plate.

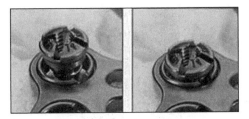

Figure 3. Left: Step 1 and Right: Step 2

© EBI. Used with permission.

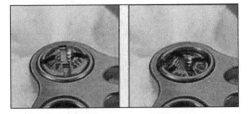

Figure 4. Left: Step 3 and Right: Step 4

© EBI. Used with permission.

Once the screw head passes under the integral ring, the screw is locked. No additional locking components are required.

8

Cervical/Thoracic Devices

Blackstone™ Ascent™ POCTS System

Blackstone Medical, Inc.

D egenerative disc disease, spinal stenosis, vertebral fracture, tumor and other disorders can affect adjacent levels of the spine. Sometimes surgical intervention is necessary to treat a spinal disorder when severe.

In complex cases that require comprehensive reconstruction from the base of the skull to the thoracic spine, the types of instrumentation systems appearing on the following pages may be considered appropriate by the spine surgeon.

Blackstone™ Ascent™ POCTS System

Blackstone Medical, Inc.

The Ascent™ Posterior Occipital Cervical Thoracic System (POCTS) is a spinal implant system. It allows the surgeon to stabilize the base of the skull (occipital region), cervical (neck), and thoracic (chest area).

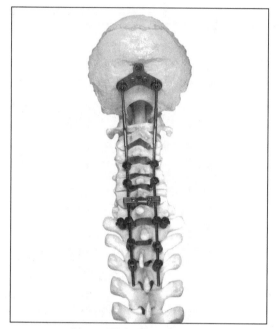

Ascent™ POCTS System

© Blackstone™ Medical Inc. Used with permission.

An important part of this system is the Monolithic Plate. This plate is implanted at the base of the skull. The plate provides a rigid and stable base from which the surgeon builds the rest of the stabilizing construct. This system is comprised of anchors, multi-axial screws, pre-bent rods, cables, and cross connectors.

OASYS™ System:
Occipito-Cervical-Thoracic Fixation
Stryker Spine

The OASYS™ System is a comprehensive fixation system used to stabilize the upper cervical ("occipito" or posterior cervical spine), cervical and thoracic spine. It has been designed to provide stability to the spine while fusion occurs.

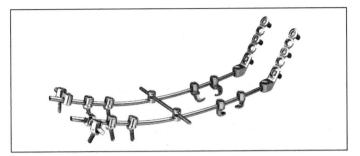

© Stryker Spine. Used with permission.

This is a low-profile modular system consisting of hooks, polyaxial screws, rods, and bone screws. Polyaxial screws have an adjustable head that allows for a high degree of screw angulation and minimizes the need to contour (bend) the rods. The low-profile design means the implant lies flatter against the spine and minimizes tissue irritation.

9

Thoracic/Lumbar/ Sacral Devices

EBI® Omega21™ Spinal Fixation System

EBI

Disorders such as degenerative disc disease, spondylolisthesis, and scoliosis may affect the stability of the adjacent thoracic, lumbar and sacral levels of the spine. Sometimes surgical intervention is required to immobilize the spine following a procedure to treat a severe spinal disorder.

In cases involving the thoracic, lumbar and sacral levels of the spine, comprehensive reconstruction may include the type of instrumentation that appears on the following pages. However, these are examples and patients should rely on the expertise of their treating spine surgeon for advice and further information.

EBI® Omega21™ Spinal Fixation System
EBI

The EBI® Omega21™ Spinal Fixation system is used to immobilize and stabilize segments of the thoracic, lumbar, and sacral spine (Fig. 1). Certain acute and chronic spinal disorders may make it necessary to surgically stabilize the spine using rods and screws.

Disorders that cause spinal instability or deformity include degenerative spondylolisthesis, fractures, scoliosis, kyphosis, spinal tumor and failed previous fusion (pseudoarthrosis).

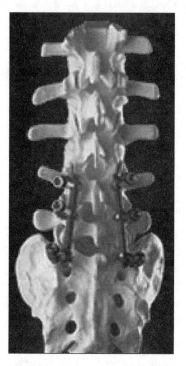

Figure 1. An Example: The lumbosacral spine has been stabilized using the EBI® Omega21™ system of rods and screws.

© EBI. Used with permission.

The EBI® Omega21™ system includes rods (Fig. 2) and specially designed screws (Fig. 3 and 4) and is used with materials (e.g. bone graft) to augment fusion. The EBI® Omega21™ system can also be used for pedicle screw fixation.

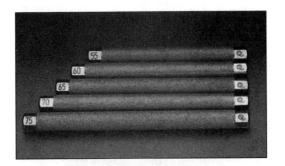

Figure 2. Rods are available in many sizes, are pre-cut, and can easily be contoured by the surgeon to fit the patient's spinal anatomy.

© EBI. Used with permission.

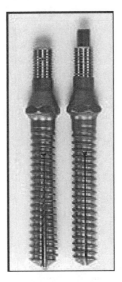

Figure 3. The EBI® Omega21™ Expandable Screw.

© EBI. Used with permission.

129

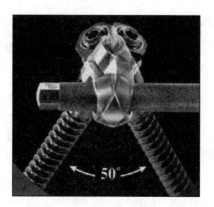

Figure 4. The EBI® Omega21™ multi-directional coupler enables screws to be implanted at different angles.

© EBI. Used with permission.

The EBI® Omega21™ system is also used with their EBI® Ionic™ Spine Spacer System.

Xia® Spinal System
Stryker Spine

The Xia® Spinal System is a comprehensive system of implants and instruments for stabilization of the spine in the thoracic, lumbar, and sacral regions. Xia® is used in the treatment of spinal instability created by degenerative disc disease, trauma, tumor, and conditions that include deformity.

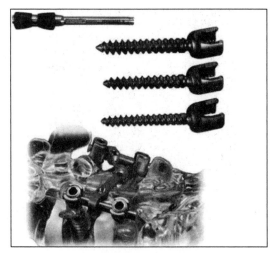

Xia® Spinal System

© Stryker Spine. Used with permission.

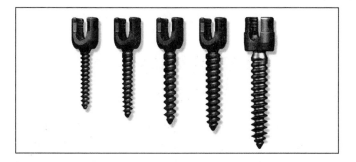

Xia® screw implants are available in several sizes.

© Stryker Spine. Used with permission.

The Xia® Spinal System is available in both stainless steel and titanium. The profile and implant volume (e.g. size) is among the lowest in the market.

10

Thoracic/Lumbar/ Vertebral Replacement Systems

EBI® Ionic™ Spacer System

EBI

S pinal fractures and tumors are examples of two disorders that may make it necessary to replace a vertebral body. The products on the following pages represent recent technological advances in devices that spine surgeons use to reconstruct the spine.

EBI® Ionic™ Spine Spacer System

EBI

The EBI® Ionic™ Spine Spacer System is designed to be used in the thoracolumbar spine; the thoracic and lumbar levels (T1 through L5). The EBI® Ionic™ spacer implants (Fig. 1) can be used to replace a diseased vertebral body, restore the height of a collapsed vertebral body, and to treat fractures. These unique spacers help to restore the biomechanical integrity at the anterior (front), middle, and posterior (rear) spinal column.

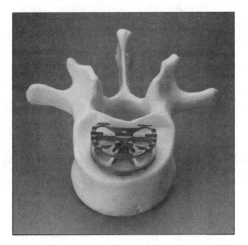

**Figure 1. The EBI® Ionic™ Spine Spacer
positioned in the middle of a vertebral body.**

© EBI. Used with permission.

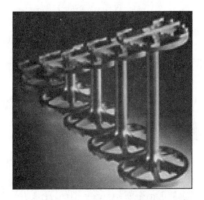

**Figure 2. The EBI® Ionic™ Spine Spacers
are available in many sizes.**

© EBI. Used with permission.

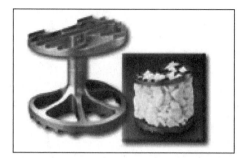

**Figure 3. The EBI® Ionic™ Spine Spacer's design
enables ease in adding bone graft.**

©EBI. Used with permission.

The EBI® Ionic™ Spine Spacer System can also be used with their EBI® Omega21™ and SpineLink® fixation systems.

Blackstone™ Construx™ PEEK VBR System

Blackstone Medical, Inc.

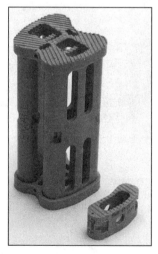

© Blackstone™ Medical Inc. Used with permission.

Blackstone Medical's vertebral body replacement (VBR) system is designed to replace vertebral bodies in the thoracic and lumbar spine (T1-L5). The size of the system's individual components allows the spine surgeon to build a construct to fit the patient.

The system components are made of PEEK (polyetheretherketon), a polymer. The material properties of PEEK include strength coupled with elasticity that is patient-friendly. PEEK is radiolucent, which means after the construct is implanted into the patient's spine, the device cannot be seen under x-ray. This affords the spine surgeon a clearer view of the spine while fusion occurs.

The MEH4™: Titanium Mesh Vertebral Body Replacement
Encore Medical Corporation

The MEH4™ is a Titanium Mesh vertebral body replacement system manufactured by Encore Medical, L.P. The product is intended to be used with other types of internal fixation systems to stabilize the spine. Pictures of the implant in various sizes are shown below.

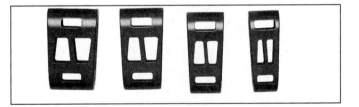

**The MEH4™ is available in different sizes
to fit the patient's anatomical needs.**

Encore Medical, L.P. Used with permission.

The interior of the mesh is open and provides a space that can be filled with bone graft material. The sidewalls of the mesh are perforated by several holes and allow for bone fusion through the sidewalls of the mesh.

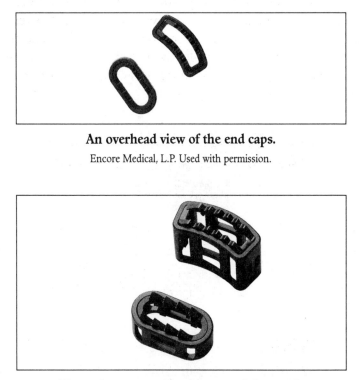

An overhead view of the end caps.
Encore Medical, L.P. Used with permission.

The end caps are placed on top of the mesh.
Encore Medical, L.P. Used with permission.

The end cap serrations, located on the top and bottom of the mesh help to provide stability and prevent movement of the implant.

NGage™ Surgical Mesh System: Sure-Footed Stabilization for the Thoraco-Lumbar Spine (T1-L5)

Blackstone Medical, Inc.

Blackstone Medical's NGage™ Surgical Mesh System is used in the thoraco-lumbar spine (T1-L5) to replace a diseased vertebral body.

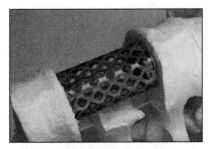

NGage™ Surgical Mesh System implanted.
Notice the device takes the place of the middle vertebral body.

© Blackstone™ Medical Inc. Used with permission.

The system includes a hollow cylindrical tube called a "lobe" and end rings both made from titanium. The walls of the tube are perforated with evenly spaced diamond-shaped openings. The openings and hollow core allow grafting material to be placed inside the device to help achieve solid fusion. This system may be used with Blackstone Medical's Spinal Fixation System.

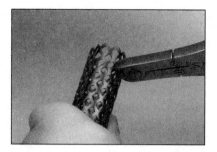

The surgeon trims the lobe to the correct length.

© Blackstone™ Medical Inc. Used with permission.

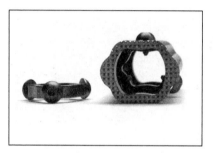

End rings feature spikes on the exterior sides that help prevent movement of the device. The standard ring stabilizes the construct.

© Blackstone™ Medical Inc. Used with permission.

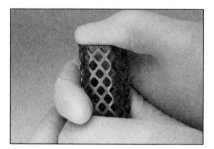

After the lobe is packed and filled with grafting material, the end rings are placed onto each end.

© Blackstone™ Medical Inc. Used with permission.

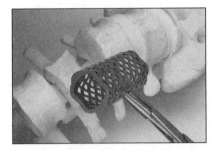

A photograph of the lobe construct as it is implanted in sawbones.

© Blackstone™ Medical Inc. Used with permission.

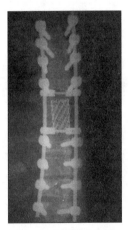

Post-operative x-ray shows the NGage™ Surgical Mesh device implanted in the patient's spine. Supplemental 'internal fixation' is also used (e.g. rods, screws).

X-Ray Courtesy Kevin Booth, MD, San Francisco, CA

© Blackstone™ Medical Inc. Used with permission.

11

Lumbar Spine Devices

Aesculap® SOCON® SRI:
Spondylolisthesis Reduction Instrument

Aesculap, Inc.

S pondylolisthesis, degenerative disc disease, and spinal stenosis are disorders that can cause low back and leg pain. The devices presented on the following pages represent new technologies that help spine surgeons to relieve symptoms and stabilize the troublesome spinal segment(s).

Aesculap® SOCON® SRI:
Spondylolisthesis Reduction Instrument

Aesculap, Inc.

Isthmic and degenerative spondylolisthesis is a common cause of lumbar symptoms and may require surgical reconstruction. Aesculap has created the SOCON® SRI to reduce spondylolisthesis with carefully controlled force and limited distraction. This remarkable device achieves reduction through levered forces applied to the L5 and S1 bodies via Aesculap's SOCON pedicle screw system.

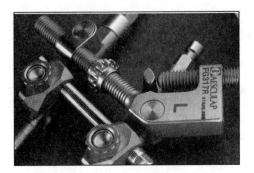

© Aesculap®. Used with permission.

DYNESYS® Spinal System
Zimmer Spine, Inc.

The DYNESYS® Spinal System is a new concept in the relief of back and leg pain caused by spinal stenosis or spondylolisthesis. The system uses flexible materials to surgically stabilize the affected lumbar vertebrae while preserving the natural anatomy of the spine. It is designed to stabilize the spine without fusion and allows some controlled spinal motion (Fig. 1 and 2).

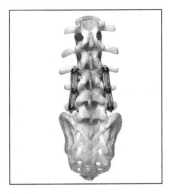

Figure 1. Front view, DYNESYS® implanted device.

© Zimmer Spine. Used with permission.

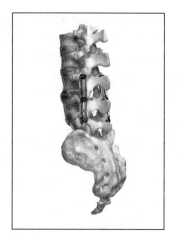

Figure 2. Side view, DYNESYS® implanted device.

© Zimmer Spine. Used with permission.

During a posterior surgical procedure, a small device is attached to both sides of the affected vertebrae. The device is comprised of spacers made of flexible plastic tubing (surgical polyurethane) surrounding a nylon-like (polyethylene) cord. The flexibility of the device is shown in Figure 3.

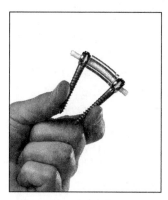

Figure 3. Close up of the DYNESYS® device.

© Zimmer Spine. Used with permission.

The device stabilizes the spinal joints thereby helping to keep the vertebrae in a more natural position and eliminates the pain caused by excess motion. The intervertebral discs and joints are kept intact. The device allows a controlled range of motion permitting bending, straightening, and twisting movements.

The DYNESYS® system is different from spinal fusion. Spinal fusion stops motion at a painful and unstable vertebral segment by permanently fusing two vertebrae together. While fusion is successful to treat back and leg pain, it eliminates joint motion and may place more pressure on adjacent spinal segments that may result in the need for further treatment in the future.

INFUSE® Bone Graft/LT-CAGE® Lumbar Tapered Fusion Device
Medtronic Sofamor Danek

Degenerative disc disease is one of the most common causes of low back pain. Sometimes spine fusion is the most effective treatment to alleviate symptoms.

Until now, spine fusion with cages required one surgical procedure to harvest pieces of bone from the patient's hip (autograft) and a second to implant the graft into the spine (autogeneous bone graft). Harvesting bone from the patient is painful and increases the risk for blood loss and other complications. Complications can add to the number of days spent in the hospital.

Bone morphogenetic protein, specifically rhBMP-2 has changed the need to harvest bone from the patient. INFUSE® Bone Graft contains a genetically engineered version of this protein (rhBMP-2) that occurs naturally.

INFUSE® Bone Graft is a powder. Prior to surgery the powder is mixed with sterile water. After mixing, an absorbable collagen sponge is soaked in the liquid solution. The sponge is used to hold a concentrated amount of rhBMP-2 at the fusion site.

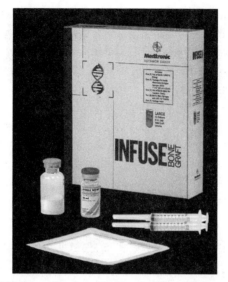

INFUSE® Bone Graft and absorbable collagen sponge.
© Medtronic Sofamor Danek. Used with permission.

INFUSE® and LT-CAGE® Work Together

The LT-CAGE® Tapered Fusion Device is a porous device made of titanium. Two devices are usually implanted side-by-side between the vertebrae. The device restores lumbar lordosis (natural spinal curvature) and maintains space between vertebrae. Before the surgeon inserts the devices into the spine, the collage sponge is rolled up and packed inside each LT-CAGE® device. The large holes in the device allows for bone formation, which leads to fusion.

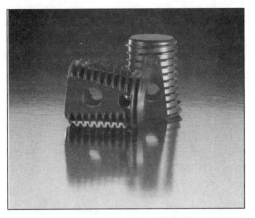

LT-CAGE® Lumbar Tapered Fusion Device.
© Medtronic Sofamor Danek. Used with permission.

LT Cage® device + INFUSE® bone graft incorporates technology developed by Gary K. Michelson, M.D.

LT-CAGE® implants and instruments incorporates technology developed by Gary K. Michelson, M.D.

Ray TFC/UNITE™ System:
Spinal Cage Devices
Stryker Spine

Spinal disorders such as degenerative disc disease and spondylolisthesis (grade one) are conditions that can create lumbar (low back) spinal instability. The Ray TFC/UNITE™ System is indicated for use in anterior and posterior lumbar interbody fusion surgical procedures.

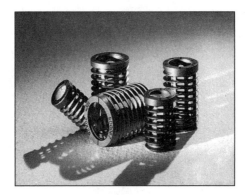

Ray TFC/UNITE™ System
© Stryker Spine—Surgical Dynamics. Used with permission.

The device is composed of titanium alloy and available in several diameters and lengths. The open-design of the device allows the surgeon to pack and fill the cage with grafting material to facilitate fusion. An optional end cap composed of ultra-high-molecular weight polyethylene may be used to cover the ends of the cage.

After the disc is removed and the disc space is prepared, typically two cages are implanted into the vacant space. The benefits include restoration of normal disc space height, nerve decompression, and spinal stability.

12

Minimally Invasive Spine Surgery

New Technology Advances Mimimally Invasive Spine Surgery: Stabilizing Screws and Rods Placed with Small Incisions, Mininal Soft Tissue Manipulation

Gerald E. Rodts Jr., MD

One of the major thrusts in spine surgery today is to develop minimally invasive procedures. By definition, minimally invasive surgery utilizes small skin incisions, minimizes the damaging effects of large muscle retraction, and attempts to leave the body as naturally intact as it was prior to surgery. The goal is to achieve rapid recovery, lessen post-operative pain, and leave cosmetically satisfying incisional scars.

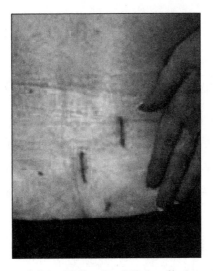

Post-Operative Incisions Following Minimally Invasive Procedure

The purpose of this article is to introduce a remarkable new technology that enables surgeons to accurately implant spinal screws and rods in fusion surgery using computer technology and minimally invasive technique.

Traditional Spine Surgery

Only a small percentage of patients suffering from chronic back and leg pain will require fusion surgery. The common indications for a fusion procedure of the low back (lumbar spine) may include slippage of the spine (spondylolisthesis), recurrent disc herniation, chronic degenerative disc disease, traumatic fracture, or other forms of spinal instability. In fusion surgery, surgeons employ bone grafts and often stabilize the spine using screws and rods.

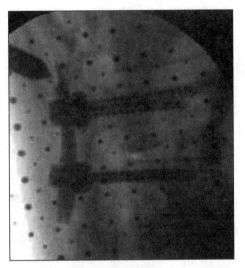

A Sample Case

Traditionally, stabilizing screws and rods are placed on the spine through an "open" approach. This means there is a standard incision, which is typically up and down in the middle of the back. The large bands of muscles in the, back are stripped free from their attachments to the spine and retracted off to each side. This allows for excellent visualization of the spine and easy access to the bones for implantation of the hardware. The downside of "open" surgery is that there can be considerable back pain from the muscle retraction, and the muscles develop some degree of permanent scar formation and damage as a result of the necessary retraction.

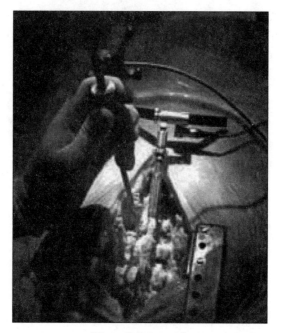

"Open" Approach

Minimally-Invasive Spine Surgery: Same Goal, Different Approach

Though the goal of implanting instrumentation (screws, rods) to stabilize the spine remain the same, minimally-invasive techniques use the power of computer-assisted image guidance to allow the surgeon to "see" the spine through the skin without making a large incision. A special type of x-ray machine called a fluoroscope has been integrated with computer technology to enable surgeons. This system is referred to as "virtual fluoroscopy" (FluoroNav™, Medtronic Sofamor Danek). FluoroNav™ allows the surgeon to locate and navigate the spine using familiar x-images in real time but with greater power and accuracy, and with only a fraction of the usual radiation exposure. When combined with new instruments designed to be placed through small incisions, this form of computer-assisted, image-guided surgery becomes quite powerful.

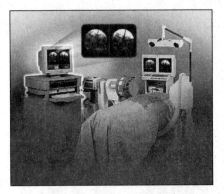

**FluoroNav™ Virtual Fluoroscopy System
(Medtronic Sofamor Danek)**

Pedicle Screws and Rods

The pedicle is a strong portion of the spinal vertebral bone that connects the front of the spine to the back of the spine. There is one pedicle on each side of each vertebral bone. Thus, placing a screw into the pedicle bone of the vertebral body proves to be a very strong way of purchasing or fixating the spine. Screws of all various designs used in this way are called pedicle screws. Once pedicle screws are placed at several levels of the spine, a rod can connect them all together on each side, giving the spine considerable extra strength.

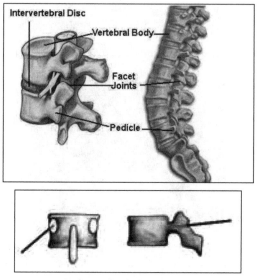

Vertebral Pedicles

One popular form of pedicle screws is made of titanium metal and has a head that can rotate to accommodate various anatomical conditions and positions. This threaded type of screw that can rotate is called polyaxial (can move about many axes). A new device called the SEXTANT™ (*Medtronic Sofamor Danek*) allows for placement of polyaxial screws and pre-cut rods to be delivered to the spine through the skin. Open procedures with long skin incisions can be avoided. The SEXTANT™ device is what delivers the polyaxial screws along a trajectory provided by FluoroNav™ (computer-assisted image guidance).

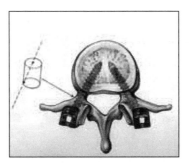

Pedicle Screws Implanted

When a screw is placed through a very small incision in the skin, it is called a percutaneous procedure. Using the SEXTANT™ device, the surgeon navigates the spine using images provided by the FluoroNav™ device and places screws straight through the skin, fat, muscle and finally into bone. The screws are placed without disturbing the natural connections of muscle and tendons to bone.

The SEXTANT™ device prepares a path through these tissues by bluntly dissecting through and creating a path. Then, a specially cut rod is passed through this path right into the heads of the screws. Using virtual fluoroscopy (FluoroNav™), each step of the procedure is "visualized" but without radiation exposure. The screw-rod connection is then tightened, and the SEXTANT™ device is removed. The patient is left with a stronger spine thanks to the stabilizing screws and rods, but all that is visible on the outside are a few small incisions the size of a fingernail.

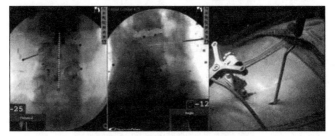

Extension of Virtual Instrument beyond Skin Surface

Benefits

The initial experience with SEXTANT™ and FluoroNav™ have proven that it is a safe, effective way to implant spinal instrumentation that achieves the same result as open surgical placement of rods and screws. The following, however, are clearly emerging as benefits of percutaneous procedures over the conventional open operation:

(1) Surgical incisions are less painful.
(2) Blunt muscle dilation and dissection leaves the anatomy more natural than muscle release and retraction.
(3) Blood loss is reduced with percutaneous procedures.
(4) Scars are cosmetically superior.
(5) The hospital stay is shortened.

Conclusion

Post-operative studies have clearly proven the efficacy, accuracy and reliability of the SEXTANT™. Surgeons and patients nationwide are recognizing the power of computer-assisted, image-guided surgery done with the minimally invasive approach.

CD HORIZON® SEXTANT™
Multi-Level Rod Insertion System
Medtronic Sofamor Danek

Medtronic Sofamor Danek's SEXTANT™ Multi-Level Rod Insertion system is a Minimal Access Spinal Technology (MAST). This technology enables rods and pedicle screws to be implanted at multiple levels in the spine using minimally invasive surgical techniques.

During a minimally invasive surgical procedure, the surgeon operates through small incisions made in the skin. Sometimes these procedures are called percutaneous, which means through the skin. The possible benefits to the patient include reduced tissue trauma, no need for muscle stripping, less blood loss, reduced post-operative pain, shortened hospitalization, quicker recovery, and smaller scars.

At the heart of the SEXTANT™ Multi-Level Rod Insertion system is the mechanical device pictured below. Through two small skin incisions, this mechanical arc-type device accurately implants the rods and pedicle screws to stabilize the spine.

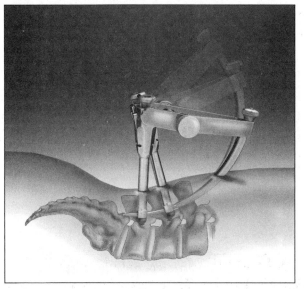

Percutaneous Rod Insertion Set.

© Medtronic Sofamor Danek. Used with permission.

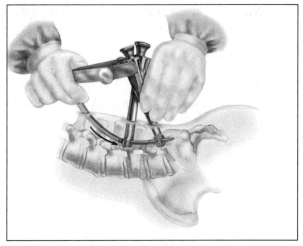

Surgeon passes the rod through the screw heads.

© Medtronic Sofamor Danek. Used with permission.

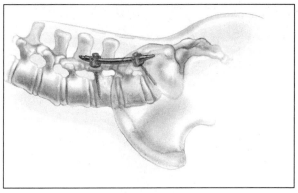

Lateral (side) view of the lumbar spine
demonstrating the rod and pedicle screw construct.

© Medtronic Sofamor Danek. Used with permission.

The SEXTANT™ Multi-Level Rod Insertion system enables spine surgeons to accomplish the same outcome without an extensive open surgical approach. Patients are spared tissue trauma, post-operative pain, and a large scar.

158

Minimally Invasive Spine Surgery Lumbar Discectomy: A Patient's Perspective

Richard G. Fessler, MD, PhD
Robert E. Isaacs, MD
Laurie Rice-Wyllie, RN, MS, ANPC

Introduction

Back pain is an unfortunate problem that will affect essentially all of us at some time during our lives. Most of the time, thankfully the problem is short lived. If it worsens to affect the sciatic (sy-attic) nerve, the pain begins to **radiate** (ray-dee-ate) down to the buttock, hip, and further down the leg. The medical term for this condition is **radiculopathy** (rah-dick-u-lop-ah-thee); an injury to a spinal nerve.

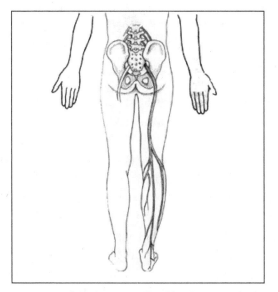

Sciatic nerve distribution

It is commonly known as **sciatica** (sy-attic-ka) or lumbago; names that bring memories of severe pain to those who have suffered from this ailment in the past. Few things hurt as badly as 'nerve pain'. Once you have felt this pain you will never forget it.

Like its cousin back pain, even the majority of ridiculer pain will end on its own without requiring surgical intervention. For the rare cases that will not heal spontaneously, surgery may lay in the future. This chapter provides an overview of ruptured discs, what can happen when a disc ruptures, why, and various treatment options for it.

What Causes Back Pain

There are a number of causes of back pain. The spine is a complex structure with a number of joints and nerves each of which is capable of producing severe pain. For this reason, generalized back pain is not only common but also very difficult to treat with directed therapy. When the pain begins to **radiate** (ray-dee-ate) down the leg a doctor can tell that a certain nerve is affected; then it is possible to direct therapy to a specific target.

The lower back is termed the lumbar spine. The lowest nerves of the lumbar spine not only make up the **sciatic** (sy-attic) nerve but are the cause for the majority of back pain that occurs. The spine not only helps to support the weight of the body but also allows for trunk mobility. This motion puts strain on the most flexible areas of the back especially the lowest two disc spaces in the lumbar spine.

The discs are spongy cushions between the bones of the spine. The discs supply mobility to the spine while protecting the bones from repeated stress. It is the constant strain that these discs take that leads to their propensity to rupture.

The disc is made of a hard fibrous shell, the **annulus** (an-you-lus) that surrounds a spongy middle, the **nucleus** (new-klee-us). Repeated stress and injury combined with weight, posture and genetics, as well as simple bad luck can lead to the nucleus rupturing through the annulus. The medical condition that results is a

herniated nucleus pulposus (her-knee-ate-ed new-klee-us pul-poe-sis, abbreviated HNP).

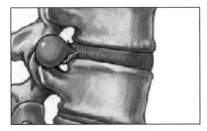

Herniated Nucleus Pulposus (HNP)
© SpineUniverse. Used with permission.

The disc spaces are named for the bones that they are sandwiched between. The **lumbar** (lum-bar) spine is made up of five bones called vertebrae, which ends at the part of the pelvis called the **sacrum** (say-krum). The disc spaces that most commonly rupture are the lowest two between the L4 and L5 vertebrae and between L5 and the sacrum. The L4-L5 and L5-S1 disc spaces are most commonly injured because, being located lowest down in a very mobile area of the spine, the most force is put on them during the course of the day.

When a disc ruptures a piece of the nucleus pushes through the annulus right where the nerve associated with that disc space lies. Because the nerve is tethered at the point in which it leaves the spine, the disc material compresses the nerve. Compressed nerves hurt. Taking weight off the spine by lying down can alleviate some of the pain. Conversely, sitting or straining, or even coughing or sneezing puts more pressure on the nerve and thereby causes more pain.

For that reason, may doctors recommend bed rest or light activity during an acute phase following a disc rupture. Pain relievers and/or muscle relaxants are used for symptom relief. Clearly some of the pain is related to inflammation around the nerve. Therefore, patients are often put on steroid packs or anti-inflammatory medications (NSAIDs such as ibuprofen). Steroids tend to help relieve pain a lot. However, because of the steroid side effects, they can only be used for a short time period. Other non-surgical treatments include **physical therapy** and direct injections of steroids near the nerve.

The vast majority of disc ruptures will heal themselves when given enough time. Therefore much of the treatment is essentially designed to alleviate symptoms while the body heals itself. Given several weeks of these treatments, most patients will be significantly better. It is the exceptional patient who remains in severe pain. When a patient's pain worsens, fails to improve, or when a patient experiences muscle weakness surgery may then be considered.

Several surgical options exist to treat lumbar disc herniation. Essentially these options are just variations of the same theme. The classic approach is lumbar **laminectomy** (lamb-in-eck-toe-me) and begins with stripping the muscle off of the back over the area of the disc rupture. A microscopic **discectomy** (dis-eck-toe-me) begins with the same step, but because a microscope is used the incision is smaller.

Over the last five years a novel approach has been developed that does not require cutting the over-lying muscles off of the bone. This approach—**MicroEndoscopic Discectomy (MED)** has been gaining favor with surgeons and patients alike. While the muscle opening is gently enlarged as opposed to cut, much of the post-operative pain is avoided. With MED, a smaller amount of bone is removed and much of the normal anatomy of the back is left intact. When all is said and done, the latter steps of all these procedures are the same—removing a small window of bone, moving the nerve and removing the ruptured disc.

MicroEndoscopic Discectomy (MED)

The patient is brought into the operating room and is put under general anesthesia. Some surgeons have chosen to perform MED under local or spinal anesthesia allowing the patient to stay awake throughout the procedure. The patient is turned onto his abdomen and padded into position. A **fluoroscope** (floor-o-scope, a machine that projects live x-ray pictures onto a screen) is brought in for use during the remainder of the operation. The patient's back is scrubbed with sterile soap and a sterile field is created. Drapes are placed accordingly and the surgery begins.

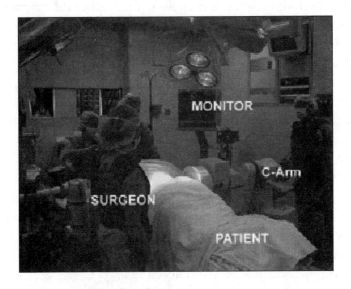

Operating Room Set Up: An example how the operating room is set up for a lumbar MED. The surgeon stands on the side of the ruptured disc. The television monitor is across the table. During the majority of the operation, the surgeon performs the surgery while watching it on the monitor.

The disc space is confirmed using the **fluoroscope** (floor-o-scope) and a long acting local anesthetic (local an-es-thet-ick) is injected through the muscle and around the bone protecting the disc. A half to one-inch incision is made. A thin wire is placed through the incision and lowered until it touches the bone.

Progressively larger dilators are brought down on top of one another following the wire. In this manner the muscle is stretched rather than cut. By the time the fourth or fifth dilator is placed, the muscles are stretched to an opening roughly the size of a nickel. It is through this opening that the procedure is performed. Over the last dilator a working channel is positioned; this circular retractor holds back the muscles and now the dilators can be removed. The retractor is held in place by a mechanical arm attached to the operating table.

Finally the **endoscope** (en-doe-scope) is attached to the edge of the working channel. The endoscope is a camera about as thick as the ink in a ballpoint pen. It projects an image of the base of the working channel blown up to the size of the TV screen. This allows for microscopic manipulation and removal of the tissues.

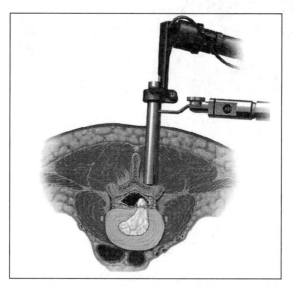

Endoscope: A representation of the working channel once the serial dilators have been removed and the endoscope is placed.

When a small amount of muscle is left over the **lamina** (lamb-in-ah) or exposed bone, this is cleaned off. In order to access the nerve, this roof of bone (the lamina) must be removed; this can be done with a small high-speed drill or small bone-biting tool called a Kerrison rongeur (wrong-ger). The bone (lamina) just below the endoscope covers the nerve as it is about to exit the spine.

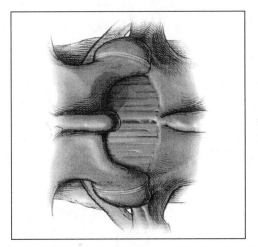

Lamina: A representation of the area of the lamina that needs to be removed to visualize the nerve and disc rupture.

© Medtronic Sofamor Danek. Used with permission.

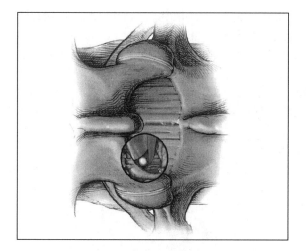

Lamina Removal: A representation of the intraoperative area and the Kerrison rongeur removing the superior (upper) lamina.

© Medtronic Sofamor Danek. Used with permission.

By removing the bony cover, the nerve can be exposed and then safely moved away. After the bone is removed, the yellow ligament (rubbery layer of tissue) can be seen which protects the underlying nerves. All the nerves except the exiting nerve are group together in the thecal sac (sheath) where they float loosely in spinal fluid.

Care is taken as the yellow ligament is separated and removed exposing the thecal sac and exiting nerve root. A very small retractor is placed just on the outside of the root and the nerve and thecal sac are moved together. Directly below the retractor lies the ruptured disc.

Ruptured disc material has a consistency similar to uncooked shrimp. When a small puncture is made into the tissue covering the disc, the disc will often times begin to ooze out. Various tools are used to remove the ruptured disc and other loose fragments of disc in the surrounding area. No attempt is made to remove the entire disc at that level—that is what is supporting those vertebrae. When completed the small hole will fill in on its own. The case at this point is essentially finished.

The wound is irrigated with antibiotics. As the scope is withdrawn, the surgeon can see the tissues coming back together. A stitch or two is placed at various levels to hold the tissues together to help healing. Typically, buried stitches are used to close the skin and non need to be removed at a later date. Commonly, Steri-Strips® (small sterile tape strips) and a loose bandage are applied to the wound. The patient is then positioned on a stretcher, woken up and sent to the recovery room. In a few hours if all goes well, the patient may leave the hospital.

Immediately After Surgery

In order to be cleared to leave the hospital, the patient must pass a few simple tests. First, the patient must be able to handle the postoperative pain on oral medications. Although not severe, there is typically some pain at the incision and some muscle ache, which will linger for a few days.

Even occasionally as the nerve regenerates there may be some twinges of pain that run down the leg along the course of the nerve. As long as these twinges do not become frequent events, they are not surprising and will get better one their own. Like incisional pain the muscular ache will persist for a few days. In fact it is not infrequent for the back to be sorer a day later. Once again, as long as it is tolerable, it will get better. Apart from pain, the nurses need to be sure that you can take care of basic functions at home. This implies that you will be able to urinate (bladder difficulty can occur after general anesthesia), walk, and tolerate food in your stomach.

What to Expect at Home

The first few days you may be more tired than usual because of the anesthesia. Your back will be tender and you may have residual leg pain, tingling or numbness. Most people will be taking medications for pain and muscle spasm. These medications are taken for approximately two to three weeks and off and on during physical therapy.

Activities and Follow-Up

We encourage you to walk as much as possible. There are many reasons walking is important. First it will begin your therapy to strengthen your legs. Walking will also help to prevent blood clots, lung congestion and increase your general feeling of well-being.

You may take a shower four days after surgery. If you have a clear dressing or gauze over your incision, this may be removed three to four days after surgery. Make sure the dressing is removed before you shower. This Steri-Strips® stay in place for one to two weeks. Eventually the strips begin to peel off on their own.

Lifting is restricted to five- to 10-pounds for at least two weeks. Using good body mechanics is very important to maintain a healthy back. You will begin formal physical therapy two weeks after surgery. The course of **physical therapy** is usually three times per week for six weeks. During your physical therapy, the therapy staff will increase your weights gradually and begin stretching exercises. You can expect some increased discomfort once you increase your activity. This should go away quickly. If it does not, you should let your physical therapist know so modifications can be made to your plan. The physical therapist will develop a home exercise program for you. Physical therapy is a crucial part of a successful outcome after your herniated disc surgery. Building strong support muscles will help ensure a health back for your future.

Most patients will see a health care practitioner at one week for a wound check and six weeks for a final follow-up. The final visit is important to assess how you are doing and answer any questions about future activity.

Conclusion

Back pain and radiculopathy (rah-dick-u-lop-ah-thee) are, unfortunately common problems that will afflict most of us at one time or another throughout our lives. Thankfully, most of these problems will be away within a few weeks. When the pain persists surgery may be an option. All surgeries directed at a disc rupture require exposing the nerve and removing the extruded disc material. The differences lie in the manner of the exposure and the postoperative pain that the patient experiences. Unfortunately, no surgery is pain free. All surgeries require a period of recovery, which may be reduced by using less invasive approaches.

METRx™ MicroDiscectomy System: The Next Step in Minimally Invasive Discectomy Utilizing the Operating Microscope

Medtronic Sofamor Danek

The METRx™ MicroDiscectomy System is a microsurgical system that uses tubular retractors inserted by way of small skin incisions to work through the normal tissue spaces that separate muscle fibers. The tubular retractors sequentially dilate the tissue spaces, which minimizes or eliminates the need for muscle stripping or cutting. The operative steps of bone removal, discectomy, and fusion are all carried out through the METRx™ tubes.

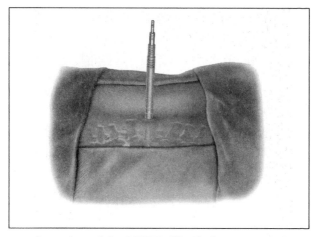

Insertion of the METRx™ tubular retractor.

© Medtronic Sofamor Danek. Used with permission.

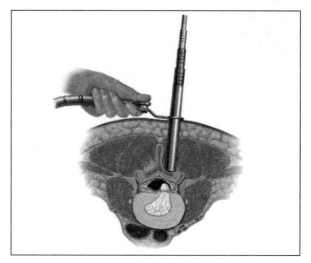

METRx™ tubular retractor separates soft tissue as the instrument is advanced to the designated spinal segment.

© Medtronic Sofamor Danek. Used with permission.

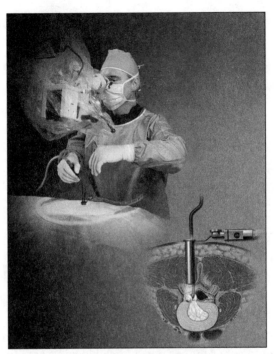

**The spine surgeon uses an operating microscope in conjunction
with the METRx™ system to perform the procedure.**

© Medtronic Sofamor Danek. Used with permission.

This type of procedure is relatively new to spine surgery. Patients
who have undergone minimally invasive micro-discectomy where
the METRx™ system was used report procedure satisfaction.

Minimally Invasive Posterior Lumbar Interbody Fusion (PLIF): A Beneficial Union

Kevin T. Foley, MD

Introduction: PLIF

Posterior lumbar interbody fusion (PLIF) is a surgical technique for placing bone graft between adjacent vertebrae (interbody). Typically, screws and rods or other types of spinal instrumentation are used to hold the spine in position while the bone heals. Indications for this procedure may include pain and spinal instability resulting from spondylolisthesis, degenerative disc disease, or when a discectomy is performed to relieve nerve compression and the patient has associated mechanical low back pain.

Spinal fusion uses bone graft to promote specific vertebrae to grow or fuse together into a solid and stable construct. Instrumentation, also called internal fixation, incorporates the use of rods, screws, cages, and other types of medical hardware to provide immediate stability to the spine and facilitate fusion.

Minimal Access Spinal Technologies

Today, spinal surgery has advanced to a new level that utilizes Minimal Access Spinal Technologies (MAST). These technologies replace traditional open surgical procedures with innovative minimally invasive techniques and tools. To grasp the importance and benefits of minimally invasive spine surgery, review the following comparison:

Open Approach

A longer incision along the middle of the back is necessary. Large bands of muscle tissue are stripped from the underlying spinal elements including the spinous process, lamina, and facets. These tissues are pulled aside (retracted) during surgery to provide the surgeon a good view of the spine and room for performing the procedure. During complex spine surgeries, these surrounding tissues (paraspinous) may need to be retracted for long periods of time. Stripping the paraspinous tissues and retracting them can contribute to post-operative pain and prolong the patient's recovery.

Minimally Invasive Approach

In minimally invasive procedures, the surgical incisions are small, there is no need (or minimal need) for muscle stripping, there is less tissue retraction, and blood loss is minimized. Special surgical tools allow the surgeon to achieve the same goals and objectives as the open surgery while minimizing cutting and retracting of the paraspinous muscles. Therefore, tissue trauma (injury) and post-operative pain are reduced, hospital stays are shorter, and patients can recover more quickly.

Open PLIF Procedure

A typical PLIF procedure involves an open incision (approximately 6-inches long) in the middle of the lower back followed by stripping the paraspinous muscles away from the spine. Bone removal (laminectomy) and lumbar discectomy are performed to remove pressure from affected spinal nerve roots.

When the offending disc is removed an empty space is left between the upper and lower vertebrae (interbody). This is filled with bone graft. Implants made of bone, metal, or other materials are typically inserted into the interbody space. Finally, pedicle screws are placed into the upper and lower vertebrae and connected with rods or plates.

MAST PLIF Procedure

Now spine surgeons can combine three innovative spinal surgical "systems" with Minimal Access Spinal Technologies (MAST)

(*Medtronic Sofamor Danek*). The combination of these systems allows a PLIF to be performed through two one-inch incisions on either side of the low back. The paraspinous muscles do not need to be stripped from the spine. The spine surgeon can perform bone removal, a discectomy, an interbody fusion, and pedicle screw insertion through the same small incisions!

METRx™ (*Medtronic Sofamor Danek*) is a microsurgical system that uses tubes inserted via small skin incisions to work through the normal tissue spaces that separate muscle fibers. These tubes are made to dilate the tissue spaces sequentially, thereby eliminating or minimizing the need for muscle stripping or cutting. The PLIF procedural steps of bone removal, discectomy, and bone graft / interbody implant placement are carried out through the METRx tubes.

TANGENT™ (*Medtronic Sofamor Danek*) is an implant and instrument system used to prepare the interbody space for insertion of precision-machined wedges of cortical bone (bone graft implants).

CD HORIZON® SEXTANT™ (*Medtronic Sofamor Danek*) is a "percutaneous" (through the skin) pedicle screw and rod insertion system. It enables the surgeon to precisely implant the screws and rods in a minimally invasive fashion. Once the METRx tubes have been removed, the SEXTANT™ screws are placed through the same small (one-inch) incisions. The rods are percutaneously inserted through tiny openings (approximately one-fourth of an inch long) in the skin. This system helps to immobilize the spine (internal fixation) so the bone grafts can heal and fuse the vertebrae together.

Conclusion

Advancements in spine surgery continue to evolve, providing surgeons with better tools and techniques to treat patients with spinal disorders. We can only expect further improvements as spine specialists continue to adopt and develop emerging technologies and integrate them into their practices.

DISC Nucleoplasty®:
Percutaneous Disc Decompression
ArthroCare Spine

For many patients, DISC Nucleoplasty percutaneous discectomy is an alternative to major spine surgery to relieve back and leg pain (sciatica) associated with a contained herniated disc (e.g. disc bulge). A contained disc herniation occurs when the disc bulges or protrudes outward, but the nucleus pulposus (gel-like interior) remains contained within the walls of the annulus fibrosus (tire-like wall).

The following pictures illustrate a normal intervertebral disc (1) and a contained herniated disc (2). A contained herniated disc causes the disc to expand beyond its normal size, which forms a bulge on one side. In Figure 2, the herniation compresses the spinal nerve, which can cause back and/or leg pain (sciatica).

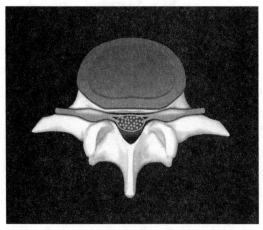

Figure 1. Normal disc.

© ArthroCare Corporation. Used with permission.

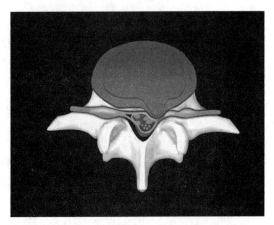

**Figure 2. Contained herniated disc bulges,
compresses the spinal nerve root.**

© ArthroCare Corporation. Used with permission.

Undergoing the DISC Nucleoplasty procedure is similar to having an epidural steroid injection. The patient is given a local anesthetic and mild sedative. Using a specialized instrument developed for use during DISC Nucleoplasty, the spine specialist inserts a needle into the center of the herniated disc. This instrument is called the Perc-D LE SpineWand™ (Fig. 3).

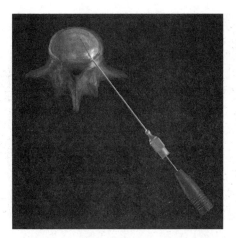

Figure 3. Perc-D LE SpineWand

© ArthroCare Corporation. Used with permission.

The needle emits radio waves that dissolve excess tissue, which reduces the size of the bulge or herniation (Fig. 4). This in turn relieves the pressure inside the disc and **decompresses** (relieves pressure) the spinal nerve root (Fig. 5). When pressure is relieved, symptoms are alleviated.

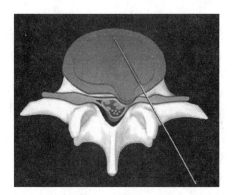

Figure 4. Perc-D LE SpineWand needle positioned to emit radio waves that dissolve excess disc tissue.

© ArthroCare Corporation. Used with permission.

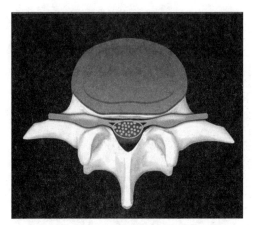

Figure 5. Pressure within the disc is relieved;
the spinal nerve is decompressed.
© ArthroCare Corporation. Used with permission.

The advantages to DISC Nucleoplasty include: the procedure is performed on an outpatient basis in less than one hour, requires only local anesthesia and a mild sedative, is less invasive and traumatic than an open spine procedure, and recovery is rapid without the need for post-operative bracing.

Patient satisfaction is high. In fact, 89% of patients who have undergone DISC Nucleoplasty report satisfaction with the procedure. The success rate is 80% and more than 35,000 patients have been treated to date with no unresolved complications.

Kyphoplasty: Treating Vertebral Compression Fractures
Kyphon, Inc.

Osteoporosis is the primary cause of vertebral compression fractures (Fig. 1). These fractures are chronically painful and can lead to progressive spinal deformity, which further impacts the patient's health and quality of life.

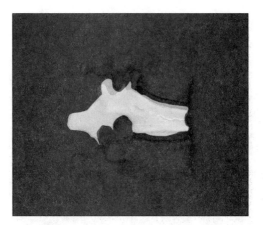

Figure 1. Fractured Vertebra, Compression Fracture

Kyphoplasty is a newer technique performed to treat compression fractures that evolved from a procedure called vertebroplasty. During kyphoplasty, a bone tamp with an orthopaedic balloon is inserted into the damaged (collapsed) vertebral body (Fig. 2). The entire procedure is performed under fluoroscopic guidance ('real time' low dose x-ray). A fluoroscopy enables the surgeon to perform the procedure minimally invasively through a small working channel.

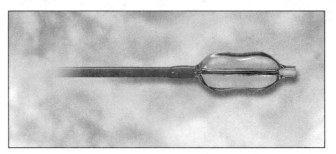

Figure 2. A close up of the KyphX® Inflatable Bone Tamp (Balloon).

Through a small incision (one centimeter), the surgeon creates a narrow pathway to the spine. After the bone tamp is properly positioned, the balloon is inflated (Fig. 3, 4). As the balloon is inflated, the shape of the fractured vertebra is restored.

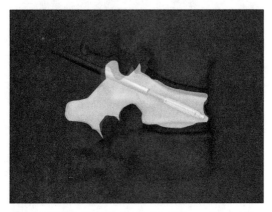

Figure 3. The bone tamp is advanced into the collapsed vertebral body with the KyphX® Balloon.

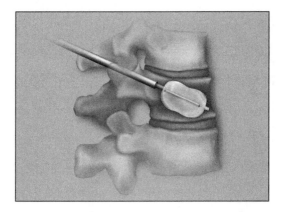

Figure 4. As the KyphX® Balloon is inflated, a portion of the collapsed vertebral body is moved restoring its original shape.

After the shape of the vertebra is restored, the balloon is deflated and removed leaving behind a cavity which is then filled with bone cement (Fig. 5, 6).

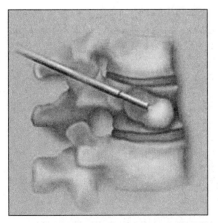

**Figure 5. The cavity created by the balloon
is then filled with bone cement.**

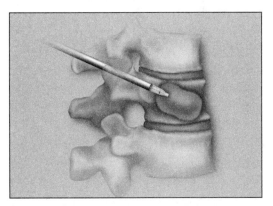

Figure 6. The bone tamp is removed and the bone cement sets.

Many studies have been conducted using kyphoplasty and patients who received this treatment have been closely followed. Patients tolerate the procedure well and report an early improvement in pain and mobility with few complications.

Kyphoplasty not only restores the vertebral body to its original height and alignment, but restores the strength and structural integrity of the bone.

The medical devices used to perform balloon kyphoplasty are manufactured by Kyphon Inc.

PathFinder™ Minimally Invasive Surgical System
Spinal Concepts, Inc.

The PathFinder™ Minimally Invasive Surgical System was developed by Spinal Concepts, Inc., a division of Abbott Laboratories. In conjunction with other surgical procedures, PathFinder™ enables the surgeon to construct a rigid supporting structure for the spine to help provide needed stability during fusion. Indicated uses for PathFinder™ include degenerative disc disease, spondylolisthesis ("shifting" of the vertebrae), and spinal stenosis (a narrowing of the spinal canal exerting pressure on the nerve roots.).

The entire PathFinder™ procedure is done through a small incision about one-inch in length. Minimally invasive surgical procedures offer patients many benefits that may include reduced pain, reduced surgical time and blood loss, shorter time in the hospital and reduced scarring.

Certain aspects of the PathFinder™ minimally invasive surgical procedure are featured below.

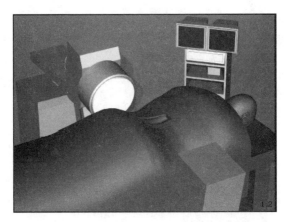

**The surgeon identifies the entry point using a
low-radiation form of imaging called "fluoroscopy."**

© Spinal Concepts, Inc. Used with permission.

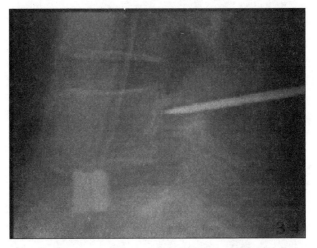

**After the affected disc space is located using fluoroscopy,
a targeting needle is advanced into the pedicle.**

© Spinal Concepts, Inc. Used with permission.

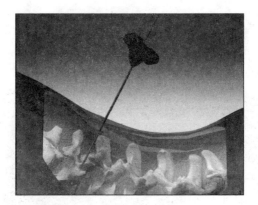

**Positioning of the targeting needle
seen inside the spine and outside of the small incision.**
© Spinal Concepts, Inc. Used with permission.

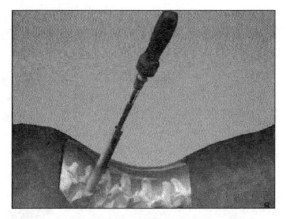

**A specialized screw with a hollow center called a cannula
is placed over a thin guide wire and inserted into the pedicle and
vertebral body. A swiveling attachment to the screw head will easily
accept a titanium rod that provides stability for the vertebral
column. The surgeon has enough flexibility to bend the rod in the
operating room to match the contours of the patient's spine.**
© Spinal Concepts, Inc. Used with permission.

Hollow tubes that temporarily attach to the screw head extend above the skin. Thin openings extending the length of the tubes allow the surgeon to guide the rod directly to the screw head and fasten the construct together.

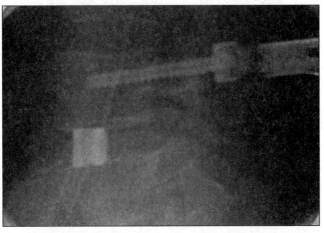

A special type of screw is placed into the pedicle.

© Spinal Concepts, Inc. Used with permission.

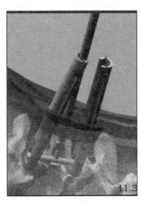

Special instruments are used to insert, position, and implant the rod. The surgeon uses fluoroscopic guidance throughout the procedure.

© Spinal Concepts, Inc. Used with permission.

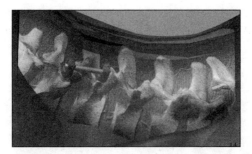

**Example illustrates a pedicle screw
and rod placement stabilizing two spinal segments.**

© Spinal Concepts, Inc. Used with permission.

13

Arthroplasty: Disc Replacement

Artificial Discs: Preserving Spinal Motion

Stewart G. Eidelson, MD

A rtificial disc replacement (ADR) is one of the most interesting topics to patients and spine surgeons. The technology behind ADR is similar to hip and knee replacement, which has proven to be successful in most patients. The idea to replace a damaged intervertebral disc with an artificial joint-type device is not new. In fact artificial disc replacement first started in Europe more than 10 years ago.

The standard surgical procedure to treat a damaged disc involves removing that intervertebral disc from between the two vertebral bodies. The empty space may be filled with cages and/or bone graft. Sometimes rods and screws are used to stabilize the spine. Once healed and fused, the motion in that vertebral segment is lost. The ADR procedure is similar and it too stabilizes the spine except spinal motion at that vertebral segment is preserved.

Currently there are several types of cervical and lumbar artificial discs in clinical trials under the guidance of the Federal Food and Drug Administration (FDA). The discs are made from the same types of materials used in artificial hips and knees; such as a polyethylene core and metal end plates. Some types of artificial discs are a metal-on-metal design (e.g. stainless steel). This technology is rapidly changing and advancing.

For more information about artificial discs,
including artificial disc clinical trial locations,
go to: *www.spineuniverse.com*

BRYAN® Cervical Disc Prosthesis
Medtronic Sofamor Danek

The BRYAN® Cervical Disc Prosthesis is a cervical (neck) intervertebral disc replacement device. The device treats stable cervical degenerative disc disease without fusion. The BRYAN® disc is designed to permit normal range of motion at the cervical spinal segment where implanted.

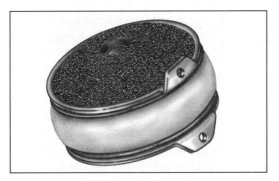

BRYAN® Cervical Disc Prosthesis
Top and Bottom: Shells
Center: Polyurethane nucleus

© Medtronic Sofamor Danek. Used with permission.

The device consists of a polyurethane core (nucleus) designed to fit between two titanium alloy surfaces (shells). A titanium porous coating covers each shell to encourage bony ingrowth and stability.

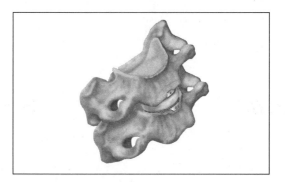

The appearance of the BRYAN® disc implanted in the cervical spine.
© Medtronic Sofamor Danek. Used with permission.

Caution: The BRYAN® Artificial Cervical Disc is considered an Investigational Device, limited by Federal (or United States) law to investigational use.

PRESTIGE® Cervical Artificial Disc Replacement
Medtronic Sofamor Danek

The PRESTIGE® artificial disc is becoming an alternative to fusion for patients with primary cervical disc disease. The PRESTIGE® disc is a metal-on-metal design made from stainless steel.

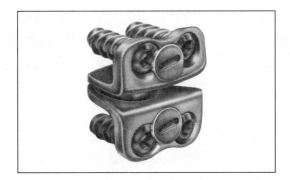

PRESTIGE® Artificial Disc.
© Medtronic Sofamor Danek. Used with permission.

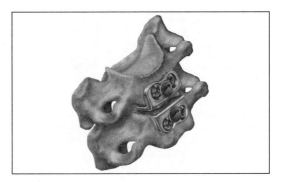

**The appearance of the PRESTIGE® artificial disc
implanted in the cervical spine.**
© Medtronic Sofamor Danek. Used with permission.

Caution: The PRESTIGE® Cervical Disc System is considered an Investigational Device, limited by Federal (or United States) law to investigational use.

Artificial Disc Replacement: Non-Fusion Technology ProDisc® Total Disc Replacement System

Synthes Spine

The ProDisc® Total Disc Replacement System is designed to replace degenerated and painful intervertebral discs of the lumbar and cervical spine. Unlike traditional fusion surgery, the ProDisc® implant is designed to maintain motion after the painful disc has been removed, and could potentially decelerate adjacent level degeneration.

ProDisc® is modular in design, with two cobalt chrome molybdenum metal endplates and an ultra-high molecular weight polyethylene inlay. When assembled, the three components create a ball-and-socket joint that closely matches the motion of the healthy spine. The endplates are attached to the vertebral bodies with a keel and have a porous coating that provides for bony in-growth and long-term fixation. The polyethylene inlay is locked into the lower endplate and contacts the highly polished surface of the upper endplate to provide a very low wear bearing surface.

The ProDisc® lumbar and cervical discs are pictured on pages 191–193.

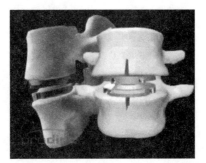

ProDisc® Lumbar Artificial Disc. Image represents the ProDisc® -L implanted in the lumbar spine.

ProDisc® (Synthes Spine, Paoli, PA, USA) Used with permission.

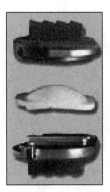

ProDisc® Lumbar Artificial Disc.
The ProDisc®-L is a modular design composed of three elements;
two endplates (top and bottom) and a core of polyethylene.

ProDisc® (Synthes Spine, Paoli, PA, USA) Used with permission.

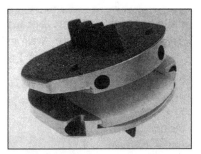

ProDisc® Lumbar Artificial Disc

ProDisc® (Synthes Spine, Paoli, PA, USA) Used with permission.

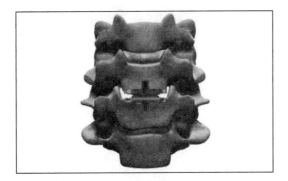

ProDisc® Cervical Artificial Disc. Image represents the ProDisc® -C implanted in the cervical spine.

ProDisc® (Synthes Spine, Paoli, PA, USA) Used with permission.

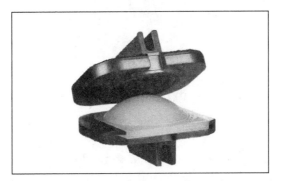

ProDisc® Cervical Artificial Disc is a modular design composed of three elements; two endplates (top and bottom) and a core of polyethylene.

ProDisc® (Synthes Spine, Paoli, PA, USA) Used with permission.

CHARITÉ Artificial Disc: First FDA-Approved Artificial Disc

DePuy Spine, Inc.

The CHARITÉ Artificial Disc is the world's first commercially available artificial disc and the first approved by the Food and Drug Administration (FDA) for use in the United States.

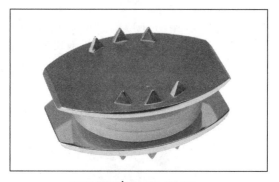

CHARITÉ Artificial Disc.

Photo Courtesy of DePuy Spine, Inc.

It is a modular prosthesis made from Cobalt Chromium alloy and Ultra-High Molecular Weight Polyethylene (a form of plastic) that incorporates a sliding core designed to restore and maintain motion of the spinal segment. With thousands of implantations worldwide since 1987, the CHARITÉ Artificial Disc has the longest clinical history of any artificial disc.

The FDA approved CHARITÉ for use in October of 2004 and is manufactured and distributed by DePuy Spine, a Johnson & Johnson Company.

MAVERICK™ Total Disc Replacement
Medtronic Sofamor Danek

Total disc replacement is becoming an alternative to spinal fusion for some patients who suffer from lumbar degenerative disc disease. The MAVERICK™ artificial disc is a metal-on-metal design made from a cobalt-chrome alloy. The artificial disc allows movement from side-to-side or back-to-front.

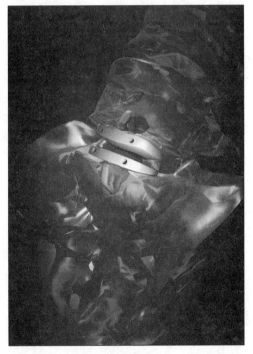

MAVERICK™ Lumbar Disc System. The artificial disc is implanted at the front (anterior) of the lumbar spine.

© Medtronic Sofamor Danek. Used with permission.

195

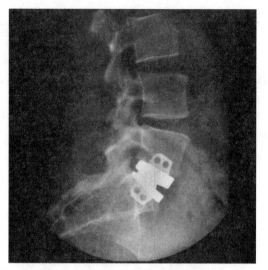

**Post-operative lateral (side) x-ray demonstrating
the position and appearance of the MAVERICK™ artificial disc
implanted between L5 and S1.**

© Medtronic Sofamor Danek. Used with permission.

Caution: The MAVERICK™ Lumbar Disc System is considered an Investigational Device, limited by Federal (or United States) law to investigational use.

14

Biological Materials

Biologic Materials: Dawn of a New Era in Spine Surgery

Jeffrey C. Wang, MD

In recent years, one of the exciting developments in the spine field has been the emergence of the use of biologic materials in spine surgery. An example is bone morphogenetic proteins (bone mor-foe-gin-et-ick proteins) or simply, BMPs. BMPs can stimulate bone growth and spinal fusion. These types of biologic materials and others are showing the potential to dramatically improve the results of spine surgery.

One of the leaders in this field is Jeffrey C. Wang, M.D. Dr. Wang is based at UCLA and, in addition to his busy practice, runs a basic science laboratory where he is constantly developing and testing new methods to treat spinal disorders. Recently, Dr. Wang gave SpineUniverse.com some of his time to help us better understand new biologic materials and the impact they will have on the future of spine surgery.

SpU: Dr. Wang, to begin, what does the term 'biologic material' mean?

Dr. Wang: A biological material is any substance that actively alters the surrounding environment and effects a change in the environment that progresses through an active, biological process. In other words, the effects are seen through increased cellular activity, growth, and differentiation.

For example, a piece of metal that is often used in a spine fusion procedure, provides stabilization which promotes fusion but, that piece of metal does not stimulate or activate cellular growth or alter cellular function; the metal is an inert material. On the other hand, a protein that attracts more cells to spine fusion can actively increase bone formation and stimulate a spinal fusion. This protein would be considered a biological material.

SpU: Are any biologics currently being used in spine surgery?

Dr. Wang: Currently, there are many biologics being used in spine surgery. This is probably the most exciting and fascinating development that has occurred in spine surgery. Common biologics in use are the demineralized bone matrices, which are extracts of human bones that biologically help to stimulate bone growth and promote spinal fusion.

Perhaps the most exciting biologics are the bone morphogenetic proteins or BMPs. These proteins are very powerful differentiation factors that can stimulate bone growth and spinal fusion. They are so effective that they can be used instead of the patient's own bone. This spares the patient significant pain, recovery time, and risks of an added procedure.

SpU: Patients are hearing a lot about BMPs. Are any being used by surgeons yet? Are the results encouraging?

Dr. Wang: BMPs are being used in human spine surgery. The FDA has approved them for use in single-level, anterior spinal fusions, when placed inside of a titanium cage.

Current studies are looking at the use of BMPs in other areas of spinal fusion. The early results of these studies are very encouraging. Since BMPs are so powerful in promoting bone formation, they are being studied for use in all areas of spinal fusion, from the neck to the lower back, and for posterior and even interbody fusions.

SpU: If my doctor plans to use autograft or allograft rather than BMP during my surgery, should I be concerned?

Dr. Wang: Patients should not be concerned if their surgeon is using allograft or autograft for their surgery. Currently, BMP is not approved for use in many areas of the spine, so the physician is actually providing the best in the standard of care. Allograft bone, especially in the cervical spine, works quite well.

Autograft bone is considered the "gold standard" and is the most commonly used graft for spinal fusion. As we study the results of BMP and other graft replacements, the use of autograft will most likely diminish, being replaced by bone graft substitutes.

SpU: Are there other biologics currently in use that you believe to be significant breakthroughs?

Dr. Wang: Definitely. Other advances that have enormous potential are the use of stem cells from a patients own bone marrow. Bone marrow cells are removed from the patient and concentrated, applied to a biologically active matrix, and then used as bone graft replacements. This synthetic, biologically active bone can be used for spinal fusion and can replace the need for taking the patient's own bone.

Gene therapy techniques are also being refined for spinal fusion and for disc regeneration. As we advance our knowledge and understanding of the biological processes that are involved in bone formation and disc degeneration, novel biological treatments are being formulated that can provide a better way to treat these spinal disorders, and treat them with less morbidity to our patients.

SpU: During the next 5 years, what other new biologic material developments do you envision?

Dr. Wang: Over the next 5-6 years, I see several biological material advances that will improve the treatment of spinal disorders. The first area lies in the newer materials that are currently being refined to replace our older, standard materials that we use today. Better metals, stronger metals, and even resorbably bioactive substances will replace current materials. New materials will be used along with some of the biological products that work in conjunction with the newer biologicals.

The next area will come with improved delivery systems for the biological materials. Because they work so well, I envision them being delivered using more minimally invasive techniques with smaller incisions, less pain, and faster recovery periods. In our laboratory, we are using image guidance and minimally invasive techniques to deliver the biological materials. The early results are very encouraging.

The last exciting development lies in extending our therapies into disc regeneration and the refinement of gene therapy techniques. Gene therapy will allow us to overcome many of the limitations of current biological restrictions and allow us to avoid fusions and preserve motion. I think this will be an exciting time for both patients and spine surgeons.

SpU: Thank you for your insights Dr. Wang. We appreciate your time.

Dr. Wang: You are most welcome.

Accell DBM100®—Bone Graft Product
IsoTis OrthoBiologics, Inc.

© IsoTis OrthoBiologics,™ Inc. Used with permission.

In some types of spine surgery where a fusion procedure is performed, bone graft is used. There are many types of bone graft including the patient's own bone (autogenous), allograft (donor bone), and demineralized bone matrix (DBM). DBM is made of bone growth stimulating proteins that have been removed or extracted from allograft bone.

IsoTis OrthoBiologics™ Accell DBM100® product is similar to putty in consistency. The product can be injected into the target area using a syringe. Since the product contains naturally occurring bone morphogenetic proteins (BMP's), it signals the patient's own bone to begin to form new bone. New bone formation is necessary for a successful fusion.

OrthoBlast II®—Bone Graft Product
IsoTis OrthoBiologics, Inc.

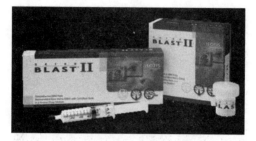

© IsoTis OrthoBiologics,™ Inc. Used with permission.

OrthoBlast II® bone graft contains demineralized bone matrix (DBM) to help stimulate new bone growth and cancellous bone to support bone formation. DBM is made of bone growth stimulating proteins that have been removed or extracted from allograft bone. Cancellous bone is the lattice-like structure inside bone.

The product is available in both putty and paste forms. OrthoBlast II® is made in a reverse phase medium, which means it is capable of being shaped by the surgeon at operating room temperature, but thickens at the surgical site from the patient's body temperature.

OsSatura TCP™—Synthetic Bone Graft
IsoTis OrthoBiologics, Inc.

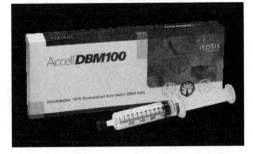

© IsoTis OrthoBiologics,™ Inc. Used with permission.

This is a synthetic bone graft product made from pure tricalcium phosphate (TCP) and resembles white granules. OsSatura TCP™ is designed to help bone to grow during the bone's natural healing process. In the body, TCP slowly dissolves and as it is assimilated, it is replaced by bone.

Trabecular Metal™ Material: An Alternative to Allograft Bone
Zimmer Spine, Inc.

Trabecular Metal™ is an alternative to allograft bone used in spinal fusion procedures. Trabecular Metal™ is a highly porous, structural biomaterial made from 98% tantalum. Tantalum is a metal in use since the 1940's for such medical applications as in skull plates after brain surgery. Since 1995, Trabecular Metal™ shapes (Fig. 1) have been used in different types of orthopaedic procedures.

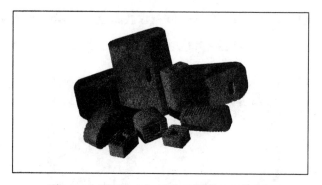

Figure 1. Trabecular Metal™ is available in different sizes and shapes.

© Zimmer Spine, Inc. Used with permission.

Trabecular Metal™ material is remarkable close to that of human cancellous bone; the same type of bone that is found near joints through the human body.

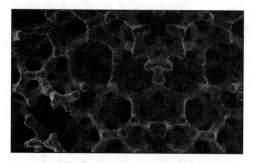

Figure 2. Trabecular Metal™ material is a structural biomaterial with bone-like properties.

© Zimmer Spine, Inc. Used with permission.

VITOSS™ Synthetic Cancellous Bone
Orthovita, Inc.

The clinical challenge in cases of bony defect due to a traumatic injury or surgery is to restore skeletal integrity. Sometimes, 'bone void filler', such as VITOSS™ is used to guide bone regeneration. The VITOSS™ microstructure is compatible with the body's cellular environment. As the body's natural healing begins, cellular activity initiates a rebuilding or remodeling throughout the structure where VITOSS™ is implanted.

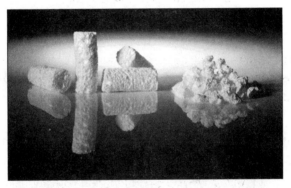

VITOSS™ is available in different shapes and forms.

© Orthovita.® Used with permission.

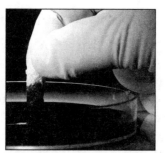

**VITOSS™ is a porous, fine-particle structure
that encourages the flow of blood and nutrients
through the entire implant, which enhances healing.**

© Orthovita.® Used with permission.

Gene Therapy: On the Cutting-Edge
Jeffrey C. Wang, MD

Gene therapy is a cutting-edge technique, which through recent advances has moved from theoretical fantasy into a potential medical therapy. It is also a powerful research and educational tool that will open the doors to a greater understanding of spinal problems. It is hoped that gene therapy will lead to the development of therapeutic treatments that could potentially solve all the problems we see in the spine.

Gene Therapy Trials

Since 1990, there have been over 300 human gene therapy trials with well over 3000 patients enrolled, and this number is steadily growing. For terminal systemic disorders such as paralysis or Parkinson's Disease, gene therapy has had limited success; however for localized conditions such as spinal fusion or disc regeneration, gene therapy can be a very powerful and successful tool.

Gene Therapy

In general, gene therapy is the transfer of genetic information into cells and tissues to achieve some desired effect. In humans, gene therapy is typically used to treat or compensate for a genetic mutation in the cellular genetic machinery or to enhance the production of a certain protein. Using gene therapy to treat systemic conditions has been quite difficult because it requires the transformation of large areas of human tissue in the body that need to last the lifetime of the patient.

For the treatment of spinal disorders however, we only need to transfer the genes to small portions of the spinal tissues and this only needs to last for a short period of time (such as for spinal fusion). Gene therapy for spinal fusion, for example, would not require that the gene be expressed or active for the life of the patient but rather only for a short period of time such as days to weeks or long enough to achieve successful fusion.

Five Basic Steps

The use of gene therapy has five basic steps, and there are a variety of methods to achieve each step.

Step 1: The gene coding for the desired protein is isolated.

Step 2: The gene is delivered to a target cell by means of a vector. This vector carries the gene and gets it into the cell.

Step 3: The cell integrates this gene and begins to produce DNA and RNA coding for the protein.

Step 4: The protein is made by the cell.

Step 5: This protein acts inside the cell or is released into the environment and then stimulates the desired action such as spinal fusion or disc regeneration.

Gene Therapy and Spinal Fusion

Spinal fusion is an excellent example of how gene therapy could revolutionize spinal surgery. Instead of putting a protein into the spine to stimulate fusion, surgeons would instead transfer the gene that codes for that protein into a portion of the spinal tissues, allowing those tissues to produce the protein responsible for bone growth. Although this seems like a complex procedure, it is much less invasive than current spinal fusion methods, which require an open incision, a certain amount of blood loss, pain to the patient and a significant period of healing. Gene therapy has the ability to dramatically change how this surgical procedure is performed. Imagine replacing an open spinal fusion surgery along with the required general anesthesia, risk of significant blood loss, pain, and prolonged recovery time, into a less invasive, one-injection procedure given on an outpatient basis without the need for a hospital stay. Although it may seem like a theoretical fantasy, in actuality there is a huge potential for the use of gene therapy in the treatment of spinal disorders.

Opening the Doors to Discovery

The main reasons for using gene therapy to treat spinal disorders would be to provide more efficient and effective ways of achieving important medical needs such as spinal fusion, disc repair or regeneration, or even regrowth of spinal cord and nerve cells. Currently we do not have answers for many of these problems; however, gene therapy can give us the methodology by which these could be potentially achieved. Studies are proving the process to be very safe and may become available in 4-5 years.

Gene therapy is still in the experimental stage and is not yet available for the treatment of spinal disorders in humans. There have been many animal studies that prove gene therapy strategies to be effective and viable techniques for achieving spinal fusion and potentially disc regeneration. In the future, the use of gene therapy will allow us to achieve better, faster and more effective spinal fusions than we can today with grafts, growth factors or proteins. Further down the line, it is likely that gene therapy will be used to accomplish disc regeneration, disc repair, spinal cord repair or even regeneration of damaged nerves.

Although not yet approved for spinal disorders in humans, gene therapy techniques will open the doors for the discovery of new and more effective therapeutics as well as allow us to accomplish treatments that today we can only imagine.

15

Braces and Fusion Stimulation

Braces Designed to Fit Patient Needs

Aspen Medical Products

Aspen Medical Products works with spine and orthotic specialists to provide patients with braces to treat many types of spinal disorders. A brace may be prescribed to be worn as part of the patient's non-surgical treatment or during post-operative recovery. Aspen offers a full line of orthotic devices used to treat disorders affecting the cervical, thoracic, lumbar and sacral spine.

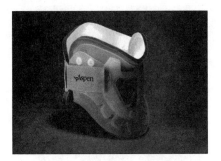

Aspen Medical Products. Used with permission.

Aspen® Cervical Collars are designed to provide support and comfort. The structure of the collar is engineered to restrict motion without causing painful pressure points.

All surfaces of the collar that come into contact with the skin are cushioned with cotton-lined, breathable foam padding. The pads are designed to draw moisture away from the skin to keep it dry and healthy.

Braces Used to Treat Many Spinal Disorders
EBI

Spine specialists prescribe braces to treat a number of conditions such as fracture, osteoporosis, scoliosis, spondylolisthesis, and whiplash. Bracing may be part of the patient's non-surgical treatment or worn after a spine surgery.

Braces are also called orthotic devices and may require fitting by a specialist. These devices come in different sizes, are adjustable, removable and are designed for comfort.

EBI offers a wide range of braces for cervical, thoracic, lumbar, and sacral spine conditions. A few of these products are presented below.

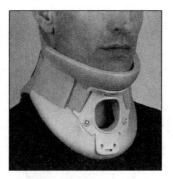

Philadelphia® Collar
© EBI. Used with permission.

EBI® Cervical Collars

The Philadelphia® Collar (above) is a traditional two-piece collar made from polyethylene foam. It provides semi-rigid support for the neck. The hole in the front of the collar is a trachea hole.

EBI® Pro-Fitt TLSO Back Brace
EBI

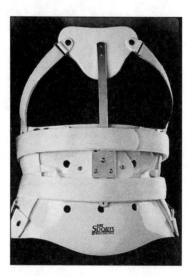

EBI® Pro-Fitt TLSO Back Brace
© EBI. Used with permission.

The TLSO back brace is prescribed to treat conditions affecting the stability of the thoracic, lumbar and sacral spinal levels (T5-S5). This brace has many straps and closings to make it easy to adjust for the right fit.

Aspen® Lumbosacral Bracing System™
Aspen Medical Products

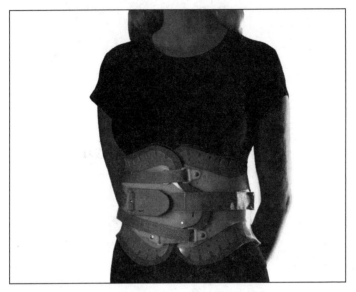

Aspen Medical Products. Used with permission.

This lumbosacral orthotic device offers patients unparalleled comfort and immobilization. The self-adjusting feature affords patients who gain or lose weight during treatment for a spinal disorder the ability to adjust the fit of the brace.

SpF® Spinal Fusion Stimulator
EBI

Since 1987, more than 100,000 SpF® Spinal Fusion Stimulators have been implanted in patients to facilitate lumbar fusion (Fig. 1). Spinal fusion is a surgical procedure that combines bone graft and instrumentation (e.g., rods, screws) to join one or more vertebrae together. This type of surgery is performed to stabilize a specific part of the lumbar spine that is causing pain (e.g., spondylolisthesis).

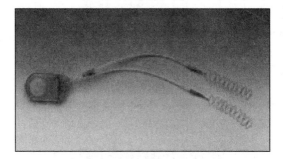

Figure 1. SpF® Spinal Fusion Stimulator

© EBI. Used with permission.

To increase the success rate for spinal fusion, a SpF® Spinal Fusion Stimulator (SpF®) is implanted during the spinal fusion surgery (Fig. 2). The SpF® is a flat, fully encased electronic device or generator based on pacemaker technology. The generator produces a safe electric current that passes through the wires that are attached to the fusion site.

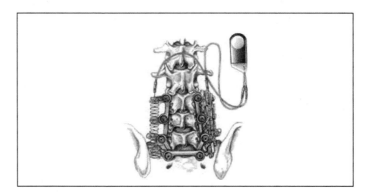

Figure 2. SpF® implanted in the lumbar spine at the fusion site.

© EBI. Used with permission.

Small electrical charges are consistently delivered to the fusion site, where the physician wants new bone to grow. These electrical charges are similar to the natural electrical charges the body emits when healing a fracture. The SpF® encourages the body to naturally produce new bone deposits to fill in the spaces around the bone graft and instrumentation.

The SpF® will stimulate bone growth for about 26 weeks. Eventually, the area becomes fused into a single bone and the device can be removed under local anesthesia through a small incision.

Spinal-Stim® Lite
Orthofix, Inc.

Spinal-Stim® Lite delivers the highest overall success rates for bone growth stimulation in spine fusion and in cases where a previous fusion has failed. Spinal-Stim's overall success has been proven in patients who are smokers, diabetics, fused using allograft (donor bone) and in multi-level fusions. In fact, the Spinal-Stim Lite is effective for up to five levels of fusion, with or without any type of instrumentation (e.g., rods, screws, cages).

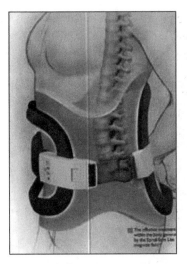

**Figure 1. Illustration shows the effective treatment
area of the Spinal-Stim in the lumbar spine.**

© Orthofix. Used with permission.

Spinal-Stim uses a technology called external Pulsed Electro-magnetic Fields (PEMF) to stimulate bone growth. During treatment, PEMF applies a time-varying magnetic field to broadly stimulate fusion (Fig. 2).

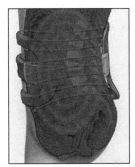

**Figure 2. PEMF enhancement of the electrical field
stimulates new bone growth and fusion.**

© Orthofix. Used with permission.

The unit is adjustable, comfortable, light-weight, easy to use and the treatment is noninvasive. The unit is designed to allow the patient unrestricted mobility.

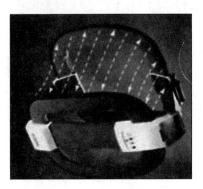

Figure 3. Front and back transducers convert energy to stimulate fusion.

© Orthofix. Used with permission.

There are no separate cables, control units or battery packs to worry about. The unit monitors treatment daily and shuts off automatically. An LED display provides instant information to the patient and physician.

16

Physical Therapy and Wellness

What Can Physical Therapy Do for Me?

Dana L. Davis, MPT, MTT

A few questions that are commonly asked a therapist include—What is physical therapy? What can a physical therapy program do for me that I cannot do on my own? How long is it going to take? Who benefits from physical therapy? What will I have to do during my therapy program? The answer to each of these questions is provided.

What is physical therapy?

Physical Therapy (PT) includes many types of conservative methods to treat, heal, and prevent injury and disability. Physical therapists primarily focus on relieving pain, promoting healing, restoring function and movement, and facilitation and adaptation associated with injury.

Further, PT focuses on ergonomics and body mechanics, fitness, wellness, and especially education. Posture, spinal stabilization, building strength in a weakened area, and injury prevention are topics covered in a PT program.

What can a PT program do for me that I cannot do on my own?

Some patients think they know how to properly exercise, manage pain and rehabilitate themselves. It is not uncommon for some patients to give therapists reasons why they do not need therapy.

For example—"I have had this before and I know what works for me" or "I know what is causing my problem because my neighbor had the same thing, so I will do what she did" and attempt to self-manage their condition.

A Physical Therapist is a specialist specifically educated and skilled in proper rehabilitation. Physical therapists receive advanced training in the management of body dysfunctions, differentiation of dysfunction from injury, and work closely with physicians to develop rehabilitation programs designed to suit the needs of each individual patient. No two PT programs are identical because no two patients are the same. Each patient's body is unique with different patterns of movement, body alignment, and habits. The physical therapist and other trained staff members monitor each patient and attempt to correct improper habits, bodily alignments, and movement patterns.

Education is one of the most important aspects in PT. Due to healthcare guidelines and reimbursement limitations, the treating physician may not have the time needed to explain what the dysfunction or injury is and its cause. The physical therapist is sometimes the person who educates a patient on the specifics of their problem, the corrective course of action, and ways to help prevent the problem from reoccurring. PT focuses on education, correction, and prevention.

How long is it going to take?

This is a popular question. Everyone has other priorities in their day and life. Exercise and therapy can sometimes seem to be an imposition. The patient has to remember that recovery from injury can be more time consuming that prevention. The severity of each patient's injury is different as is their recovery rate. In most cases, the therapist has an idea of how quickly each patient will heal within two weeks. Other factors that affect healing and recovery are the patient's compliance and dedication to PT. Therapists are healers and teachers. If the lessons taught are not practiced and learned, healing can take longer and the chance for re-injury increases.

Who benefits from PT?

Anyone who applies themselves to a PT program will benefit. As an active therapist, I work out and always observe others. I rarely come across individuals who exhibit perfect body mechanics, training techniques, or movement patterns. This is where wellness comes into play. Typically, the most appropriate patients are those who have been in accidents (e.g. work related, automobile, falls), athletes with overstress injuries, arthritic patients, pre- and postoperative patients, and others with problems related to a deconditioned body or strains.

Posture is often overlooked. Patients who make simple changes in daily habits can change their potential for injury and alleviate the current symptoms.

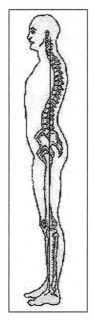

Proper posture—body alignment

Standing

When standing, think about what is comfortable. Think about what your mother told you, "Stand up straight and don't slouch!" Good standing posture involves upright positioning; shoulders back, chin neutral, abdominal muscles tight, arms in line with the body, and one foot slightly in front of the other with the knees slightly bent. This is called 'active posture'. It requires muscles to work with the skeletal system to conserve energy and protect bones and joints.

Sitting

When seated, the eyes should be level and the neck positioned so that it is not bent forward or backward. The shoulders should be level and relaxed (not slumped forward). The seat should provide appropriate support and maintain the natural spinal curves. The hips and knees should be level to each other and the ankles vertical to the knees.

Lying Down

Proper lying positions are those in which the joints are in neutral positions (neither bent excessively forward or backward). The muscles should be supported yet relaxed. Elbows, wrists, hips, and knees should be slightly bent. Too many pillows can cause the neck to 'hyperflex', which applies too much pressure to the brain's blood supply.

Poor Posture can cause forward head, rounded shoulders, excessive lordosis (humpback), posture associated with chronic cane dependants, tight and weak back muscles. Poor posture can lead to joint pain.

What will I have to do in PT?

Therapy generally includes modalities to help provide pain relief, strength and flexibility training, proper postural alignment, regaining movement and increased range of motion, improving and correcting posture, endurance training, relaxation and stress relieving techniques, balance and coordination training, proper walking, education, safety awareness, and a home exercise program.

PT is Worth Your Effort

Remember that each patient is different and therefore PT programs are individual. Be patient with yourself, your physician and physical therapy staff. Healing takes time, compliance, and diligence. If you think you can benefit from physical therapy, speak to your physician or therapist.

Physical Therapy:
Passive and Active Treatments

Susan A. Spinasanta

Physical therapy is generally categorized as either passive or active. Passive refers to treatments administered to the patient by the therapist. Active therapies are those that require patient participation, such as therapeutic exercise. Summarized below is an overview of the different types of treatments including information about posture and body mechanics.

Part 1: Passive Therapies

Electrical Stimulation (Stim) forces a muscle or muscle group to contract and relax. Physical therapists have used electrical stimulation for more than 15 years to enhance healing and alleviate swelling and pain. As the muscles are stimulated, circulation to the injured area increases. Circulation carries oxygen and nourishment to injured tissues essential to healing.

The therapist places a pair of surface electrode patches onto the skin over the treatment area (e.g. low back). Each patch is attached to a lead (insulated wire) that is connected to equipment that controls and regulates the amount of stimulation. The therapist programs the equipment to deliver stimulation for a set time period. The treatment is not painful; the patient feels a gentle pulsating or on/off sensation.

Heat and Ice Therapy

Heat increases circulation and decreases stiffness, muscle spasm, and pain. Physical therapists apply moist hot packs wrapped in several layers of toweling to deliver deep heat. Unlike a heating pad that only delivers surface heat, moist heat penetrates deeply into soft tissues and stimulates local circulation more than heat alone. Heat is not applied immediately following injury, as heat increases muscle inflammation. **Ice** decreases pain by slowing the speed of nerve impulses. Inflammation, the body's vascular response to injury may subside when cold therapy is applied. Cold reduces the temperature of tissue beneath the skin. Cold packs, ice massage, and iced towels are usually recognized as first aid during the initial 72 hours following trauma. Application of cold therapy for an extended period of time can harm the skin. Treating with ice should be supervised by a physical therapist, especially when treating an overworked body part.

Hydrotherapy is probably one of the oldest therapeutic treatments. Hydrotherapy is similar to a whirlpool bath or Jacuzzi®. Whirlpool tanks come in different sizes and some are large enough to accommodate the entire body. Similar products are portable and can be added to a bathtub.

During hydrotherapy the water temperature, direction of the jets, and water intensity are controlled to maximize the benefits. Warm water hydrotherapy is not recommended immediately after injury as heat increases muscle inflammation.

Myofascial Release improves circulation, decreases muscular tension, and increases range of motion. Myofascial release is a form of localized massage that affects the muscle **fascia** (fay-sha). Muscle and groups of muscle are encased in sheets of fascia. During myofascial release the fascia is manipulated by hand to systematically stretch the tissue. Scar tissue or tight tissue may be loosened using cross friction hand motions during massage therapy.

Ultrasound is a common and effective way to increase circulation to a specific area, stimulate healing, calm muscle spasm, and break down unwanted scar tissue. High frequency sound waves are generated from the head of the ultrasound wand and transmitted through a gel that is applied to the skin before treatment. The treatment is soothing.

Physical Therapy:
Passive and Active Treatments
Susan A. Spinasanta

Part 2: Active Therapies

Aquatic Therapy

Many patients with osteoarthritis (os-t-o-arth-rye-tis) have found exercising in water to be beneficial. A pool offers a gravity-free environment that allows the patient to perform simple exercises without stressing painful joints. Movement increases circulation to the joints and can help relieve stiffness. Some patients have found swimming to be a good exercise that helps to loosen up stiff joints and strengthen muscles.

Movement and Conditioning

Therapeutic and conditioning types of exercise are supervised by the physical therapist who teaches the patient how to properly move within a pain free range. This does not mean that exercise will be easy in the beginning. Remember the saying, 'anything worthwhile is worth working for'.

Warming-Up the Body is the First Step

Sometimes warm-up activities include riding a stationary bike followed by light stretches. The type of warm-up and therapeutic exercise is dictated by the patient's individual treatment program designed by the therapist. Temporary muscle soreness 24 to 48 hours following exercise therapy is normal and should be expected. As exercise becomes more regular discomfort will subside.

Stretching Helps to Increase Flexibility

Resistive and strengthening exercises may be added as the patient progresses. Some patients are not able to move the injured area without assistance. In these cases, the physical therapist manually moves the injured area (e.g. arm leg) to increase range of motion.

Home Exercise Program

A physical therapy program usually includes a home exercise program designed to meet the patient's individual needs. The home exercise program may include written instructions and illustrated movements as a guide. Before starting or changing an exercise program, consult the therapist first. If necessary, changes can be discussed with the patient's physician.

Physical Therapy:
Passive and Active Treatments

Susan A. Spinasanta

Part 3: Posture and Body Mechanics

Proper posture combined with good body mechanics helps to minimize spinal stress and prevent back and neck injury. The importance of posture and body mechanics is stressed during physical therapy and may be one of the first lessons a patient learns.

Good posture means the shoulders are held slightly back and level, the ears are in line with the shoulders, the chin is tucked slightly inward, and the pelvis is shifted forward allowing the hips to align with the ankles. Notice in the illustration below how the plumb line hangs directly from the ear lobe down the middle of the arm to the ankle.

227

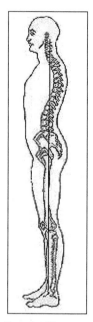

Proper Posture

How does movement affect the spine?

To demonstrate, the least amount of pressure or stress is applied to the spine when lying flat on the back. As a person stands upright, the stress climbs to 3 times and when seated 4 times. The stress rises 5 times as a medium-weight box is lifted.

The stress level can double when poor body mechanics are involved in movement. For example, bending at the waist instead of the knees to pick a lightweight item up off the floor can cause 10 times the amount of unnecessary stress to the spine.

When poor posture and body mechanics are habitual and repetitive, the risk for trauma increases. The following prevention suggestions may help you to avoid painful injury.

Avoid Stressful Work Habits

- Avoid leaning over the desk for a prolonged time periods.
- Sit close to the work area in a seat with good back support.
- Adjust the chair height so the knees are bent at a 90-degree angle when seated.
- Rest the elbows on the work surface at a 90-degree angle.
- Avoid cradling the telephone against an ear and shoulder.

Lifting and Carrying Tips

- First, take a look at the object to be moved. If it looks too heavy or cumbersome, find help.
- Plan the pathway before beginning to move the object. Remove obstacles in the pathway before lifting the object.
- Think about how to maintain good posture and body mechanics during the event.
- Get as close to the object as possible. Place the feet slightly apart and flat on the floor. Bend at the knees to provide a stable base of support.
- Tighten the stomach muscles, keep breathing and smoothly lift the object using the muscles in the arms and legs—not the back.
- Try to hold the object at the sides and bottom. Keep the object close to the body with the back straight and carry the object with the elbows slightly bent.
- When you carry shopping bags or luggage, split the load in two. Try to carry the same amount of weight in each hand.

Push or Pull?

- Pushing is usually more efficient. Keep the back straight and use the knees to push. Stay close to the object by repositioning the body from time to time.

Reaching Tips

- Consider the size, weight, and location of the object.
- Use a stable stool or ladder to face the object as close as possible. Stand on the stool or ladder with flat feet. One hand can be used for additional support.
- Avoid looking overhead to prevent neck strain.
- Consider storing often needed items within easy reach without the need for a step stool or ladder.

EBIce® Cold Therapy System
EBI

An essential part of a patient's postoperative treatment includes pain management. Cold therapy and medications are often prescribed following spine surgery to help control pain, inflammation and blood loss. The EBIce® is a portable cold therapy system that provides rapid cooling to the surgical or injured site through a sterile pad (Fig. 1). A small hand-held device enables the patient to control the amount of cold water that circulates through the pad (Fig. 2).

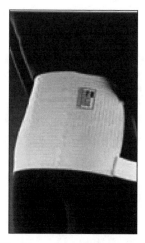

Figure 1. Treatment applied at the low back.

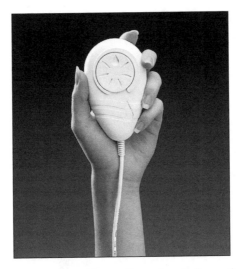

Figure 2. Control is at the patient's fingertips.
© EBI. Used with permission.

The EBIce® system is better than an ice bag because it lowers the skin temperature more consistently and evenly, and is comfortable. Patients give the product high marks and attribute it to helping them to recover more quickly from their spine surgery by decreasing pain and swelling.

The EBIce® Cold Therapy System includes applications for other body parts such as the ankle, foot, shoulder, knee, and hand. Many patients have used the system both before and after surgery, and before a physical therapy session.

The STABILIZER™ Pressure Biofeedback
Chattanooga Group

This simple device is used to provide feedback to ensure quality, and precision in exercise performance and testing. The device monitors the position of the low back and provides feedback to the healthcare professional and patient when the abdominal muscles are not actively or effectively protecting the spine.

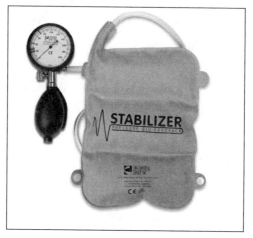

The STABILIZER™ Pressure Biofeedback device.

© Chattanooga Group. Used with permission.

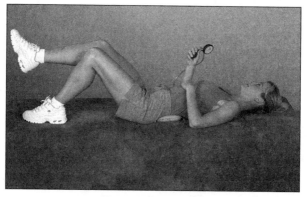

An example of how the device is used.

© Chattanooga Group. Used with permission.

Orthotrac™ Pneumatic Decompression Vest
Orthofix, Inc.

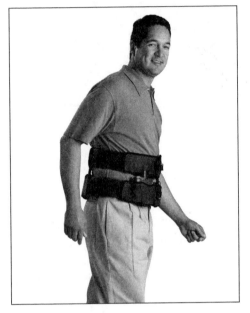

© Orthofix. Used with permission.

Braces have been used for years to help relieve back pain. Now a new type of device is available that utilizes technology adapted from engineering science. This new device is the Orthotrac™ Pneumatic Decompression Vest (Fig. 1).

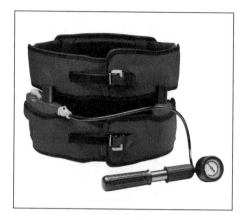

Figure 1. Orthotractm Pneumatic Decompression Vest
© Orthofix. Used with permission.

Unlike conventional braces, the Orthotrac™ vest is equipped with small pneumatic lifting devices that transfer 30% to 50% of the body's weight from the lumbar spine onto the pelvic bones. The pneumatic unloading technology is designed to relieve mechanical low back and/or leg pain. Mechanical low back and related leg pain changes as the body repositions during activity. This type of pain can be caused by disorders including herniated discs, pinched spinal nerves, foraminal spinal stenosis, degenerative disc disease, spondylolisthesis, and osteoporosis. The effect of unloading the lumbar spine is similar to standing in shoulder-deep water. Patients report significant pain relief when wearing the Orthotrac™ vest.

As with other treatments and therapies, not all patients with mechanical low back pain are suitable candidates for a successful outcome. Patient selection is very important. The Orthotrac™ vest is available by prescription and is not intended to be worn all day. Rather the vest provides patients temporary pain relief thereby enabling participation in physical therapy and muscle-strengthening exercise. Many patients have been able to return to a more active lifestyle including work.

Tempur-Pedic Swedish Sleep Systems®: Good Night's Sleep without Back and Neck Discomfort

Tempur-Pedic International, Inc.

A high-tech alternative to innerspring mattress design is a pressure-relieving material called TEMPUR®. It is the core material in the design of Tempur-Pedic's Swedish Sleep Systems. TEMPUR is unlike any other memory material used in other sleep systems today. The TEMPUR material conforms to an individual's unique shape and distributes pressure evenly. As the material conforms to the body's shape, the neck and spine are anatomically supported.

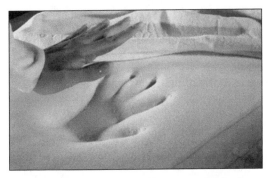

TEMPUR material conforms to the body.

© Tempur-Pedic.® Used with permission.

The attributes of the TEMPUR material is provided by Tempur-Pedic:

The viscoelastic characteristic of TEMPUR pressure-relieving material allows it to return to its original shape after being forced to change under the pressure exerted by your body. The material seems to know exactly how far to let you "sink in" so that every point on the contour of your body is supported—and then amazingly "flows" back to its original shape when you get up.

235

To put it into visual perspective—the following pictures illustrate how the Tempur-Pedic Swedish Sleep System® supports the spine.

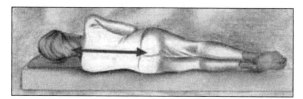

**The Tempur-Pedic® Swedish Mattress™
conforms to and supports the entire body.**

© Tempur-Pedic.® Used with permission.

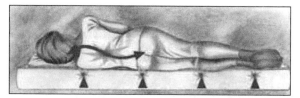

**Conventional mattresses do not support the
spine or body correctly and may create painful pressure points.**

© Tempur-Pedic.® Used with permission.

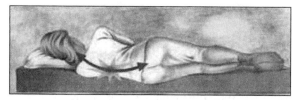

**Sleeping on a waterbed may not provide adequate support leading
to "the hammock effect", which is not conducive to a healthy spine.**

© Tempur-Pedic.® Used with permission.

Tempur-Pedic's Swedish Sleep System® is just that—a system that includes their mattress and foundation or adjustable base.

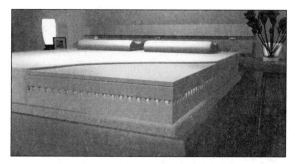

A cut-away picture of the Tempur-Pedic® Swedish Mattress™
© Tempur-Pedic.® Used with permission.

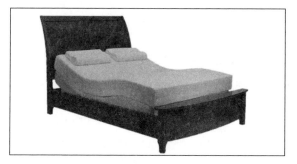

The Tempur-Pedic Adjustable Swedish Sleep System®
© Tempur-Pedic.® Used with permission.

Tempur-Pedic® offers many types of sleep systems, neck pillows, lumbar supports, seat wedges, and products to help make travel more comfortable.

Zero-Gravity Products to Ease Back Pain
Relax The Back

One of the greatest contributing factors to neck and back pain is the position of the body when sitting, sleeping, and reclining. To help prevent and alleviate neck and back pain, the spine must be properly positioned and supported. An important aspect to preventing and relieving back pain is the principle of Zero-Gravity.

Zero-Gravity occurs when the torso is properly angled with the thighs and lower legs positioned above the heart. In this position, the amount of pressure exerted onto the spine is greatly reduced. When the spine is positioned at Zero-Gravity, full body muscle tension is relieved and circulation is improved. It is a completely stress-free position. The principle of Zero-Gravity is an important part in the design of many Relax The Back™ products.

BackSaver Zero-Gravity Bed Wedge System

This product is a unique bed wedge system that can be arranged in a variety of comfortable and relaxing positions. The wedges can easily be converted to allow the person to sit upright or in the Zero-Gravity position (below).

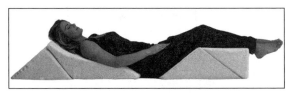

© Relax The Back.™ Used with permission

Zero-Gravity Perfect Chair

This chair comes with an integrated lumbar support, generous seat and leg room, easy-adjust position control, articulated headrest, and a patent-pending guide rails system for smooth reclining.

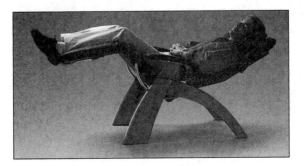

© Relax The Back.™ Used with permission

ContourSleep by Relax The Back™

The mattress is topped with a 3-inch layer of ventilated pressure and temperature sensitive memory foam that can be customized using interchangeable plush or firm inserts. The ventilated foam chambers promote airflow as the body moves to regulate body heat and dispel moisture for a cooler night's sleep. A ventilated natural latex insert is an option for people who prefer a more traditional foam mattress.

Beneath the pillow top are multi-density layers of high resiliency foam including a layer of AirCool™ foam that is profile cut to further enhance air circulation. The mattress is constructed from an acrylic fiber called Allergy Care with an organic chemical additive called Triclosan proven to be effective against bacteria. The fibers are self-replenishing to prevent indoor allergens caused by common dust mites.

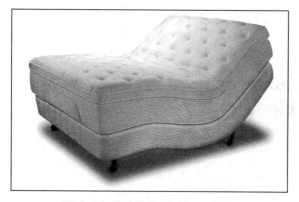

© Relax The Back.™ Used with permission

In the picture above, the ContourSleep by Relax The Back™ is shown available with a fully adjustable foundation that allows it to be moved into hundreds of relaxing positions including Zero-Gravity at the touch of a button. Other options include dual massage for back and legs.

17

Pain Management

Pain Management Techniques to Help Conquer Back and Neck Pain

Steven H. Richeimer, MD

Back and neck pain is one of the leading causes of lost work time, second only to the common cold. It affects 65-85% of the population of the United States at some point in their lives.

The most common cause is sprain, strain, or spasm usually brought on by poor lifting techniques, improper posture, or an unhealthy ergonomic environment. Another common cause is disc problems brought on by injury, wear and tear, or age. Other causes include spinal stenosis (spinal sten-oh-sis), osteoarthritis (os-t-o-arth-rye-tis), osteoporosis (os-t-o-pour-o-sis), and other conditions discussed in this book and at www.spineuniverse.com.

Pain management often takes a multidisciplinary approach to minimize or eliminate pain. The goals include increasing physical activity, eliminating unsafe medication use, and learning lifestyle behaviors that work toward wellness. The purpose of this chapter is to help you to understand pain management. Included is an explanation of the different types of pain and treatments pain management specialists use to fight pain.

Types of Back and Neck Pain

Acute Pain (ah-cute pain) can be defined as severe short-term pain. Post-operative pain is an example. Acute pain is self-limiting, which means the pain acts to warn you to cease or limit activity that could cause additional tissue damage. The more intense and prolonged an acute pain episode is, the more likely it will lead to chronic pain. This makes sense given the information that we are beginning to learn about how the central nervous system changes in response to intense pain. As a result of intense pain, neurons in the spinal cord that help to prevent pain transmissions actually die. At the same time, pain-transmitting neurons grow more connections to other nerves, become more sensitive, and react more strongly to painful stimulus.

The study of neuroplasticity (nu-row-plaz-te-city), or how the nervous system changes and molds itself, is one of the hottest new areas in neuroscience. It seems to be the basis for the processes of learning and memory. It appears however, that the nervous system not only learns useful information but also 'learns' or remembers pain leading to the development of chronic pain.

Chronic Pain. Rather than being the symptom of a disease process, chronic pain is itself a disease process. Chronic pain is unrelenting and not self-limiting. It can persist for years and even decades after the initial injury. There are many factors that affect the development of chronic pain such as age, level of disability, depression, or the presence of nerve damage.

Neuropathic Pain (nu-row-path-eck pain) is usually described by patients as burning, electric, tingling, and shooting in nature. Often this type of pain cannot be controlled using traditional pain killing oral drugs. Management of neuropathic pain may include other medications (that are often not thought of as pain medicines) and multiple treatment modalities such as physical therapy, physical rehabilitation, relaxation training, trigger point injections, epidural steroid injections, sympathetic blocks, spinal cord stimulators, intrathecal morphine pump systems, and various surgical techniques.

Nociceptive Pain (no-si-sep-tive pain) is localized pain, which is usually described by patients as sharp, aching, or throbbing. Post-operative pain, pain associated with trauma, and arthritic pain are examples of nociceptive pain. Nociceptive pain usually responds to non-steroidal anti-inflammatory drugs (NSAIDs) and opioids (oh-pe-oids, strong prescription pain killers).

Pain Management Treatments and Therapies

Anti-Depressant Medications. There is considerable evidence that tricyclic anti-depressants are effective for the treatment of a variety of pain conditions such as migraine headache and neuropathic pain.

Non-Steroidal Anti-Inflammatory Drugs (NSAIDs) are valuable analgesics (pain relieving medications). These drugs do not alter the patient's cognitive functions, cause respiratory depression, or nausea. However, NSAIDs are associated with significant side effects especially with long-term use.

Epidural Steroid Injections (ESI). The traditional epidural (ep-e-do-ral) steroid injection technique involves the physician feeling the patient's spine in order to guide the placement of the needle between the spinal vertebrae. A newer technique involves using x-ray fluoroscopy to guide the needle directly into the neural foramen; the point where the affected nerve root exits the spinal canal.

Injections of steroids into the lumbar epidural space are particularly useful to alleviate pain that radiates from the lower back into a leg. This pain may be caused by disc herniation or spinal stenosis, which triggers nerve root irritation, inflammation, and pain. Similarly, ESIs are used to treat neck pain that extends into the arms.

Facet Joint Injections involve the injection of steroid medication into the affected spinal facet joint (fah-set joint) to reduce inflammation and pain. Injections into these joints or blocks of the nerves that feed the facet joints can often be very helpful to relieve pain. This problem is more common in the lumbar spine, but does occur in the cervical spine too.

Trigger Point Injections are muscle blocks. Muscles chronically tense or in spasm become tender and painful. The pain triggers more spasm that can develop into a vicious cycle. Injections into the muscle can help to break the cycle.

Nerve Blocks are injections of medication onto or near nerves. The medications that are injected include local anesthetics, steroids, and opioids. Blocks are used to control acute pain (e.g. shot at the dentist or an epidural block for the surgical delivery of a baby). X-ray fluoroscopic guidance is sometimes used for accurate needle placement.

Blocks can provide periods of dramatic pain relief, which promotes the desensitization of sensory pathways. Steroids can help reduce nerve and joint inflammation, and the abnormal triggering of signals from injured nerves. Further, blocks are used to provide diagnostic information such as helping to determine the pain source.

Peripheral Nerve Blocks affect the peripheral nerves; nerves beyond the brain and spinal cord. These nerves transmit sensation and motor (movement) signals.

Sympathetic Nerve Blocks. Chronic pain conditions often involve sympathetic nerve malfunctions. These nerves regulate blood flow, sweating, and glandular function. For example, blocks administered in different areas of the spine help to reduce pain that involves the face, arm, hands, legs, and feet.

Physical Therapy (PT) addresses body mechanics (posture), building strength and flexibility through exercise, injury prevention, and utilizes many modalities. Modalities include electrical stimulation, heat and ice therapy, hydrotherapy, ultrasound, and massage.

Biofeedback is used to treat many types of conditions including chronic pain, migraine headache, spinal cord injury, and movement disorders. It is a type of relaxation training and behavior modification. Biofeedback works to control physiological reactions such as muscle tension, body temperature, heart rate, brain wave activity, and other life responses. The therapy requires the patient's intense participation to learn how to control these functions. Biofeedback does not work for all patients.

Electrical sensors, attached to monitoring equipment, are applied to special points on the patient's body. The monitoring equipment feeds back the patient's progress. The biofeedback therapist teaches the patient mental and physical exercises, visualization, and deep breathing to treat their specific disorder (e.g. low back muscle spasms).

Procedures

Intradiscal Electrothermoplasty (IDET) is an unproven minor procedure used to treat low back pain. Back pain and sciatica can be caused by degenerative disc disease, which may include disc bulging or herniation. These conditions can cause nerve impingement, inflammation, and pain. During IDET and under x-ray guidance, a needle is inserted into the affected disc. A special wire is then threaded through the needle into the disc. After the wire is properly positioned, it is heated. The goal of the procedure is to destroy the small nerve fibers that have invaded the degenerated disc. IDET causes the annulus (disc wall) to partially melt. This is turn triggers the body to grow new protein fibers to reinforce the annulus.

Radiofrequency Discal Nucleoplasty is similar to IDET. It is a newer procedure. A needle is inserted into the disc. Instead of a heating wire, a special radiofrequency probe is inserted through the needle into the disc. The probe generates a highly focused plasma field with enough energy to break up the molecular bonds of the gel in the nucleus essentially vaporizing some of the nucleus. The result is that 10-20% of the nucleus is removed, which decompresses the disc and reduces the pressure both on the disc and the surrounding nerve roots. This technique may be more beneficial for sciatic-type pain than IDET, since nucleoplasty can actually reduce the disc bulge pressing on the nerve root. The high-energy plasma field is actually generated at relatively low temperatures minimizing the danger to surrounding tissues.

Pumps and Stimulators

Patient-Controlled Analgesia (PCA) is used to treat postoperative pain. The device is equipped with a pump that is attached to the patient's intravenous line (IV). It is programmed to dispense the correct dose of pain-relieving medication directly into the bloodstream. The patient is given control over pain by operating the PCA with a hand-held push-button mechanism.

Once past the acute pain stage, the patient is switched to oral medication. The doses administered by PCA are smaller and available more frequently. Pain relief is consistent. This helps to prevent sleepiness and weakness allowing the patient to ambulate sooner. It has been proven that PCA reduces the overall amount of medication needed to control pain.

Spinal Pumps are called **intrathecal** (intra-thee-cal) spinal pumps. Intrathecal refers to the fluid containing space that surrounds the spinal cord. The benefit of administering pain relieving medication through a spinal pump is that medications taken orally are diffused throughout the entire body. A spinal pump delivers pain-relieving medication precisely where it is needed. This treatment is considered after standard conservative treatments have been ineffective or have caused intolerable side effects.

The pump is surgically implanted beneath the skin of the patient's abdomen. A catheter is run to the level of the spine from where pain is transmitted. Medication is pumped directly into the spinal fluid allowing for a much more potent effect on the spinal cord. This drastically cuts down on the amount of medication needed and provides better pain relief with fewer side effects.

The pump is refilled every 1-3 months by inserting a needle through the skin and into a diaphragm on the surface of the pump. Several different medications can be administered this way. Since the system is beneath the skin, the risk of infection is minimized and the patient can be fully mobile and active.

Spinal Stimulators. Instead of medication to relieve pain, spinal stimulators use electrical pulses on the surface of the spinal cord to reduce pain. The stimulators are similar to pumps in that they are surgically implanted beneath the skin but differ in that electrical signals are used to ease pain.

Electrical signals are passed through the tip of the catheter at the precise location near the involved segment of the spinal cord. The result is a tingling over the painful area, which eases pain. Current theory is that the electrical current input alters the spine's processing of the pain so that the patient's pain is reduced. The patient is able to control the stimulator by holding a magnetic pulsing device over the skin on top of the implanted generator disk. The stimulator appears to be effective for patients with back and leg pain that spinal surgery did not relieve. There is data that shows that these patients will do better with the placement of a stimulator than they will with repeat surgery.

Conclusion

As we learn about neuroplasticity, we have learned that good pain management starts with prevention. When possible, physicians should strive to reduce the intensity and duration of acute pain. When pain does persist, then a multidisciplinary approach is often most effective. In severe cases, when pain does not respond to usual treatments, then the more invasive techniques such as nerve blocks, spinal pumps, and spinal stimulators should be considered.

It is not always possible to cure the cause of pain—but it is usually possible to reduce pain and suffering.

An Integrated Approach to Back and Neck Pain
Geraldo Zloczover, MD

Integrated pain management is a new approach to treating acute and chronic back and neck pain. Pain afflicts millions of patients suffering spinal stenosis (spinal sten-oh-sis), degenerative disc disease, osteoporosis (os-t-o-pour-o-sis), failed back surgery, facet disease, myofascial pain, and degenerative scoliosis (sko-lee-oh-sis).

Today patients find that modern medical professionals have a different view of pain. Chronic pain is no longer considered long lasting acute pain and pain perception is individual to the patient.

Traditional spine care and pain management specialists have merged to form collaborative programs for the comprehensive treatment of pain. Patients find many advantages to these programs including the centralization of medical care with less duplication of services from different medical disciplines. An integrated pain management program educates the patient to understand their pain and to learn how it can be controlled. The patient and specialist work together as partners to determine the best treatment.

Pain Assessment

A pain management assessment begins with the patient's pain history, which includes the location, intensity, and duration of pain as well as factors that alleviate or aggravate pain. A physical and neurological examination is performed. Further, the patient's medical history and test results are reviewed including radiographs (e.g. x-rays, MRI).

Multidisciplinary Approach

A multidisciplinary approach means the patient's pain program may include different types of treatment. Treatment is provided by the medical professional that specializes in a specific type of treatment. Medical professionals may include a pain management specialist, physical therapist, rehab specialist, and occupational therapist.

Conservative non-surgical treatment may include a combination of pain relieving medications, anti-inflammatory drugs, physical therapy, and injections. Alternative therapies include acupuncture, biofeedback, stress reduction, and diet modification. In this chapter different types of injection therapies are presented.

Epidural Steroid Injections

Steroid injections are potent anti-inflammatory agents injected directly into the epidural space located close to the affected nerve roots. The epidural space is the area surrounding the spinal cord and nerve roots. These injections are most effective in the presence of nerve root compression. Scientific studies demonstrate inflammation of the spinal nerves following prolonged compression leads to irritation and swelling.

These injections are most effective when given during the first weeks after the onset of pain. Usually two or three injections one to two weeks apart are required. Only one injection is given when complete pain relief is achieved. The number of injections is limited to a maximum of three to avoid systemic side effects from the steroids. Side effects are minimal and consist mainly of mild tenderness in the injection area, which disappears in one to two days.

Sterile Procedure

Epidural steroid injections and nerve blocks are administered in a hospital or outpatient medical facility under sterile conditions. Through an IV (intravenous line), the patient is given medication to relax. Numbing medication is injected into the skin area where the injection will be placed. The physician uses **fluoroscopy** (floor-os-co-pee) to guide the needle into the epidural space at the appropriate spinal level (cervical, thoracic, lumbar). After the procedure, the patient is moved into the recovery area and monitored for about an hour.

Nerve Blocks are injections of anesthetic, steroid and/or opioid (oh-pe-oid) medications. Nerve blocks are performed to relieve pain and/or to determine if a specific nerve root is the pain source. Anesthetic (an-es-tha-tick) medications numb the nerves, steroids are potent anti-inflammatory drugs that reduce swelling, and opioids are powerful drugs that fight pain. In some cases, nerve blocks can provide extended periods of pain relief. Some of the different types of nerve blocks are listed below.

Cervical, Thoracic, Lumbosacral Medial Branch Blocks target the medial branch nerves. Medial branch nerves are very small nerves that communicate pain from the spine's facet joints (fah-set joints).

Facet Joint Blocks are performed to reduce inflammation and pain and to confirm that a particular facet joint is the pain source. The facet joints are small-paired joints on the back of the spine that help to provide spinal stability and guide motion in the back.

Selective Nerve Root Blocks are performed to reduce inflammation and pain and to determine if a specific nerve root is the pain source.

Conclusion

During the last decade, pain management has evolved into an integral part of patient care, which has dramatically affected the medical community. Medical professionals have a better understanding of pain. Attitudes are changing, diagnostic protocols have advanced, technology has improved procedures, and there are more medication options. The horizon continues to brighten for patients who suffer pain.

Drug Preparations Applied to the Skin Help Relieve Pain
Stewart G. Eidelson, MD

Topical pain-relieving drugs are preparations applied to the skin as a cream, ointment, gel, or spray. Topical "drug" applications are used to help reduce inflammation below the skin surface and alleviate nerve pain. Some of these drugs are available only with a doctor's prescription and others can be purchased over-the-counter (OTC).

Spine specialists may recommend the use of a topical pain-reliever to help relieve the symptoms of **osteoarthritis** (os-t-o-arth-rye-tis), **rheumatoid arthritis** (room-ah-toyed arth-rye-tis), neck or low back sprain/strain, **whiplash,** muscular and joint pain, and some types of nerve pain. Two common types of topical pain relievers are local anesthetics (an-es-tha-ticks) and analgesics (an-all-jee-siks).

- Local anesthetics are substances used to reduce or eliminate pain in a limited area of the body. These work by blocking the transmission of nerve impulses. One type of local anesthetic combines lidocaine and prilocaine (EMLA®). It numbs the skin for a period of two to three hours and is helpful to reduce pain prior to injection or insertion of an intravenous line (IV).
- Analgesics are non-steroidal anti-inflammatory drug (NSAIDs) preparations in cream, ointment, or gel form. Topical analgesics are used to reduce swelling and ease inflammation that can cause pain.

Over-the-Counter Products

The use of topical pain-relieving agents is not a new concept. Products such as Lanacane® or Solarcaine®, both available OTC, have been used for years to treat minor sunburn, abrasions, and cuts.

BenGay® and IcyHot® are examples of OTC drugs used to help relieve joint pain commonly associated with arthritis. These preparations work primarily as local anesthetics without analgesic compounds added. Aspercreme®, Sportscreme®, and Myoflex®—available OTC, contain a type of salicylate; a chemical substance similar to, but not aspirin.

Topical Analgesics

Newer types of topical pain-relieving creams, ointments, and gels have become available and contain NSAIDs such as ibuprofen and dilofenac (Voltaren® Emugel). These topical preparations work to reduce swelling and inflammation of soft tissues (tendons, ligaments, muscles) caused by trauma or disorders such as osteoarthritis and rheumatoid arthritis.

Capsaicin

Another type of topical preparation contains Capsaicin (Zostrix®, Dolorac®). These prescription preparations work by reducing the levels of the chemical substance P, which is involved in transmitting pain impulses to the brain.

Important Considerations

Whether the topical preparation to be used is purchased OTC or prescribed, keep in mind the substance is a drug. That is why it is important that the patient discloses their medical history, including prescription, OTC, supplements (e.g. vitamins, herbs), and allergies to their treating medical professional.

Other medical conditions may affect the use of a topical pain-relieving medication. These conditions include:

- Broken or inflamed skin, burns, open wounds.
- Atopic dermatitis or eczema (skin disorders).
- Glucose-6-Phosphate Dehydrogenase (G6PD) deficiency (a type of anemia).
- Severe liver or kidney disease.
- Methemoglobinemia (defective iron in the red blood cells; inhibits oxygen delivery to tissues).
- Intolerance to certain oral medications.
- Asthma.

Safe and effective use of a topical pain-relieving agent involves many of the same considerations as if taking an oral medication.

(1) Take the time necessary to review the package insert.

(2) Use as directed or prescribed.

(3) Do not apply topical pain-relieving preparations to open wounds, burns, broken or inflamed skin.

(4) Avoid applying near the eyes, lips, mouth, and ears.

(5) If accidentally swallowed, contact a poison control center, doctor or hospital immediately.

(6) If a rash, side effects, or allergic reaction develops, contact the treating physician at once.

Conclusion

When used appropriately, topical preparations can help reduce or alleviate pain caused by osteoarthritis, rheumatoid arthritis, and soft tissue trauma. Patients whose pain is relieved using topical agents require lower doses of oral medications. This means they can avoid many of the harmful side effects associated with oral drugs.

Drugs Used to Treat Pain: Opioids—Narcotics
Steven H. Richeimer, MD

There are many different types of drugs used to treat back and neck pain. These drugs include narcotics and non-steroidal anti-inflammatory drugs (NSAIDs). Although the terminology is not precisely correct, pain-relieving **opioids** (oh-pe-oids) are often called **narcotics**, and they may be prescribed to treat acute pain (ah-cute pain) (severe, short-lived pain), post-operative pain and certain types of chronic pain. Sometimes the treating physician will prescribe an NSAID with a narcotic to relieve pain associated with **inflammation** (in-flah-may-shun).

Taking pain medication is a serious decision and the patient should be aware of the possible side effects from a single drug taken as well as the dangers of combining different medications. This is a decision that should be made with the treating physician who knows the patient's medical history.

The purpose of this article is to help patients understand what an opioid narcotic is, how they work, the common side effects, and drug induced symptoms that may warrant medical attention.

Opioids: Powerful Narcotic Drugs

Opioids (oh-pe-oid) have been used for centuries to relieve pain. Those opioids that are derived from the seedpod of the poppy plant (papaver somniferum) are referred to as opiates (oh-pe-ates). Morphine and codeine are commonly known opiates derived from opium. Other opioids include synthetics such as meperidine (Demerol) and chemicals naturally found in the body, such as endorphin.

How Drugs Treat Pain

Opioids work to relieve pain in two ways. First, they attach to opioid receptors, which are specific proteins on the surface of cells in the brain, spinal cord and gastrointestinal tract. These drugs interfere and stop the transmission of pain messages to the brain. Second, they work in the brain to alter the sensation of pain. These drugs do not take the pain away, but they do reduce and alter the patient's perception of the pain.

Factors Affecting "Effect"

The effects of any drug depends on the amount taken at one time, the patient's past experience with the drug, and whether the drug is injected, administered intravenously or taken orally. The patient's psychological and emotional stability may also affect the effect of the drug. Of course, combining drugs with other opioids or alcohol can produce profound side effects. Some side effects can be harmful or lethal.

Tolerance

Chronic opioid use may result in a tolerance to the drug. This means that higher doses of the drug are needed to obtain the same initial pain relieving effects. Some patients develop a cross tolerance, which means prolonged use of one opioid may cause a tolerance to develop to all opioids.

Common Side Effects

All drugs cause side effects. Some are acceptable and others are bothersome or even dangerous. Common side effects include euphoria, drowsiness, nausea, vomiting, constipation, dilated pupils and respiratory depression. The patient should always report side effects to the treating physician.

Withdrawal

The body adapts to the presence of an opioid. Withdrawal symptoms appear when drug usage is reduced or abruptly stopped. Symptoms of withdrawal may begin as early as a few hours after usage is dramatically lowered, and the symptoms peak two to three days thereafter. Never alter the prescribed dosage or stop an opioid without the treating physician's knowledge and advice. Withdrawal symptoms include a craving for the drug, restlessness, moodiness, insomnia, yawning, abdominal cramps, diarrhea and goose bumps.

Conclusion

Pain is personal—no two patients perceive pain in the same manner. This is one reason why patient/physician communication is important to manage pain effectively. There are hundreds of drugs and other treatments available to treat back and neck pain. Managing pain does not have to be a solitary effort when patients and physicians work together.

Pain Management and Spinal Cord Stimulation

Advanced Neuromodulation Systems, Inc.

Many patients living with chronic pain that is difficult to manage now have new options for pain management. ANS (Advanced Neuromodulation Systems) has developed devices that can help control pain. Neurostimulation (use of a spinal cord stimulator) delivers low-levels of electricity directly to nerve fibers. This direct approach to treating chronic pain at the source can be very effective in modulating or lessening pain.

There are two types of spinal cord stimulators; an Implantable Pulse Generator (IPG) and Radio Frequency (RF). To see if the patient is a candidate for spinal cord stimulation (SCS), they undergo a "trial" or testing period. The trial period helps the patient to determine if SCS is the best treatment option. If SCS works well for the patient, then a permanent system is implanted via a minor invasive surgical procedure.

The IPG's power source consists of a battery and electronics housed in a single metal container. The IPG is implanted under the skin. The leads are placed above the spinal cord (epidural space) and connected to the IPG (Fig. 1).

Figure 1. Genesis® Implantable Pulse Generator (IPG) SCS System

© Courtesy of Advanced Neuromodulation Systems. Used with permission.

The Radio Frequency (RF) spinal cord stimulators are similar to IPGs. One difference is the RF's power source (battery) is situated outside of the body; it uses an external power source. The transmitter sends radio waves through the skin to an implanted receiver. The receiver in turn sends mild electrical energy to the leads (Fig. 2).

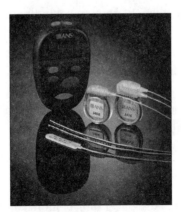

Figure 2. Renew® Radio Frequency SCS System

© Courtesy of Advanced Neuromodulation Systems. Used with permission.

There are many factors that affect whether a patient is a good candidate for spinal cord stimulation. These include the patient's medical history and type, severity, and location of pain.

Spinal Cord Stimulation: Is it Right for You?

Edgar G. Dawson, MD
Mary Claire Walsh

In the wide world of pain-relief treatment options, one that has been successful for many chronic back pain sufferers is spinal cord stimulation. In this therapy, electrical impulses are used to block pain from being perceived in the brain. Instead of pain, the patient feels a mild tingling sensation.

How Does Spinal Stimulation Work?

A small wire (called a lead) connected to a power source is surgically implanted under the skin. Low-level electrical signals are then transmitted through the lead to the spinal cord or to specific nerves to block pain signals from reaching the brain. Using a magnetic remote control, you can turn the current on and off, or adjust the intensity. The sensations derived from the stimulator are different for everyone; however, most patients describe it as a pleasant tingling feeling.

There are two kinds of systems available in spinal cord stimulation. The more commonly used system is a fully implanted unit that utilizes a pulse generator and a non-rechargeable battery that must be replaced over time. The second system relies on radio frequency and includes a transmitter and an antenna, which are carried outside the body (much like a pager or cell phone) and a receiver, which is implanted inside the body.

Your physician will help you determine which system is better for you based on your condition, your lifestyle, and how much electrical energy is required to provide you with adequate pain relief.

Who is a Good Candidate for Spinal Stimulation?

This therapy is not for everyone. Generally, spinal cord stimulation may be considered when:

a) Conservative treatments have not been successful.
b) Surgery is not likely to help.
c) The patient has no untreated drug addictions.
d) The patient has had a psychological evaluation.
e) The patient does not have a pacemaker or other contraindications.
f) The patient has had a successful trial period with the spinal cord stimulator.

First Step—The Trial Period

Before a spinal cord stimulation system is permanently implanted, most physicians recommend a trial period. During this time, a temporary stimulator is surgically implanted to allow you to try the therapy for a while (a minimum of 24 hours, but can be up to several weeks). This trial period is important to determine if the therapy provides satisfactory pain relief and is a good way to find out if you are comfortable with the sensations of spinal stimulation. If the system works for you, a permanent stimulation system can be implanted.

Next Step—Implantation

Using a local anesthetic to numb the area, the surgeon will insert the wire lead through a needle or through a small incision. Once the lead has been implanted, the stimulation system will be activated and you will help the surgeon determine how well the system works on your pain.

The lead is connected to a receiver, which is implanted under the skin usually in the buttocks or abdominal area. However, other areas of the body can be used if these are not comfortable for you. Depending on your body shape and size, the receiver should not be easily visible through the skin.

You can expect some pain and swelling at the incision site and in the area where the receiver is implanted. This is normal and should only last a few days. Your doctor may prescribe a pain relief medication to help during this time.

Immediately following implantation, you should avoid lifting, bending, stretching, and twisting. However, light exercise, such as walking, is encouraged to build strength and help relieve pain.

Risks and Benefits

As with any surgical procedure, there are risks, including:

- Infection
- Bleeding
- Headache
- Allergic Reaction
- Spinal Fluid Leakage
- Paralysis

In addition, there are some risks that are specific to the spinal cord stimulator. These may include:

- Stimulation stops or only works intermittently
- Stimulation occurs in the wrong location
- Over-stimulation
- The lead could move or become damaged (this may require surgical repositioning or removal)
- Poor system connection

However, there are also numerous benefits to using this type of therapy, including:

- Spinal cord stimulation allows you to be in control of your pain relief—you decide when it is needed
- Since the system is portable, you should be able to resume all of your usual daily life activities at home and at work
- You can travel, since your pain relief travels with you (keep in mind that sitting for long periods of time can increase pain)
- You will be able to participate in most recreational activities such as walking, swimming, and gardening
- Alleviating some or all of you pain will have a positive effect on your mental outlook, decrease stress, and improve your overall quality of life

Things to Keep in Mind:

Since spinal cord stimulators utilize electric impulses as well as magnets, there are a few precautions users must keep in mind, including:

1) Do not drive or use heavy equipment while the stimulator is activated. However, you can use the stimulator if you are a passenger.
2) Spinal cord stimulators may set off metal detectors (such as in airports). You will be given special identification that certifies you have a spinal cord stimulation system. Be sure to carry this with you to get you through these checkpoints.
3) Anti-theft devices (such as in retail stores) may temporarily increase stimulation if your system is on when you walk through. This will not harm the system, but may not be pleasant for you. It's usually best to turn off the stimulator before walking through any of these devices.
4) When flying, airline personnel may require you to turn off the stimulator during take off and landing.

5) Normal household equipment, such as cell or portable phones, computers, TVs, microwaves, and other appliances are safe to use with the stimulator. The stimulator should not cause any interference with these items.

6) The magnet on the stimulator control device may cause damage to certain items or erase information on items with magnetic strips such as bank or credit cards, video or audiocassettes, and computer disks. The magnet can also stop watches and clocks, so you may want to store the magnet at least two inches away.

Is it Right for You?

While there is no guarantee that spinal cord stimulation will alleviate all of your discomfort, most patients report a 50%—70% decrease in pain. This decrease can make your pain much more manageable and allow you to return to a more active life. Not everyone can benefit from this therapy; however, it might be worth a visit to your spine specialist to see if you are a good candidate.

EBI® VueCath® System: Spinal Endoscopic Tool for Diagnosis and Treatment
EBI

The VueCath® System is a fiberoptic endoscope developed for use by a spine or pain management specialist to see the inside of the lumbar space to treat patients with chronic low back pain (Fig. 1). Sometimes low back and leg pain is caused by inflammation or compression of a spinal nerve due to a disc injury (e.g., herniated disc), postoperative scarring, narrowing of the spinal canal (e.g., spinal stenosis), or other abnormalities.

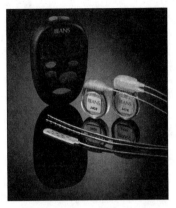

Figure 1. The VueCath® Endoscopic Tool.
© EBI. Used with permission.

As a diagnostic tool, the VueCath® system aids in the diagnosis of inflammation or scarring around a spinal nerve when other tests (e.g., MRI) are inconclusive. As a treatment tool, VueCath® enables the specialist to see the inside of the spinal canal and to inject medications precisely where needed to treat the cause of pain. The endoscopic catheter (flexible tube) is very small; about the diameter of a pencil lead.

The outpatient procedure is performed in hospital or clinic under local anesthetic. Intravenous sedation can be added if necessary. The procedure takes from 15 to 30 minutes. The soft steerable catheter is inserted near the tailbone (Fig. 2).

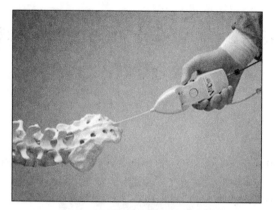

**Figure 2. The flexible 'steerable' catheter
is inserted near the tailbone.**

© EBI. Used with permission.

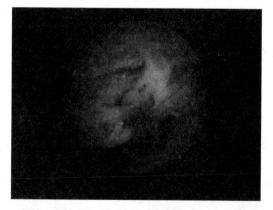

**Figure 3. A real-time view inside the spine. A sample of
what the spine specialist can see using the VueCath® System.**

© EBI. Used with permission.

During the entire procedure, images of the spinal canal are dis-
played on a video monitor (Fig. 3). The procedure is not painful.
Some patients have reported feelings of pressure in the back or legs
or tingling sensations. Patients are released home shortly after the
procedure and usual activities can be resumed the following day.

Glossary and Pronunciation Guide

Acute Pain (ah-cute): Severe or sharp short-lived pain that may follow injury or surgery.

Allograft (al-o-graft): Cadaver donor bone.

Analgesic (an-all-jee-sik): Pain medication.

Anesthesiologist (an-es-thee-z-al-oh-jist): Physician who administers sedatives and pain medication during surgery.

Ankylosing Spondylitis (AS) (an-key-low-sing spon-dee-lie-tis): Chronic, progressive inflammatory disease affecting the spinal joints.

Ankylosis (ak-key-low-sis): Disease that causes the spine to lose flexibility and stiffen.

Anterior (an-tear-e-or): Front.

Anterior Longitudinal Ligament (an-tear-e-or long-ji-tude-inal): Spinal ligament that attaches to the front of each vertebra.

Anti-Depressant (anti-dee-press-ant): Prescription medication to alleviate depression and anxiety.

Anti-Inflammatory (anti-in-flam-ah-tory): Over-the-counter (OTC) or prescription drug to reduce inflammation, swelling.

Annulus Fibrosus (an-you-lus fye-bro-sis): Tough tire-like outer layer of an intervertebral disc.

Arachnoid (ah-rack-noid): One of the protective membranes covering the spinal cord.

Arthropathy (arth-row-pathy): Joint disorder.

Arthritis (arth-rye-tis): Common joint disease that causes inflammation and pain.

Articulate (ar-tick-you-late): Joint movement.

Artificial Disc: Spinal disc replacement. Similar to hip and knee joint replacement. Also called Artificial Disc Replacement (ADR).

Autogenous Bone Graft or Autograft: Patient's own bone used in a spinal fusion procedure.

Benign (be-nine): Non-cancerous.

Biopsy (by-op-see): Removal of a tissue sample either surgically or by other means (needle aspiration).

BMP: See Bone Morphogenetic Protein.

Bone Density Scan: Also called a Bone Mineral Density Scan (BMD). Diagnostic test to measure bone density, strength.

Bone Graft: Bone harvested from the patient or a bone substitute used in spinal fusion.

Bone Morphogenetic Protein (BMP) (bone mor-foe-gin-et-ick protein): Bone growth stimulating proteins used in spinal fusion.

Bone Stimulator: Device used to stimulate bone growth.

Bony Overgrowth or Bone Spur: Abnormal bone growth, also called an osteophyte (os-t-o-fight).

Brace: Custom-fitted, removable support worn to stabilize the spine or curb abnormal curve progression.

Bulging Disc: A Contained Disc disorder, part of the annulus of an intervertebral disc protrudes, the nucleus remains contained.

Burst Fracture: Vertebral body breaks apart.

Cage: An interbody cage or device implanted between vertebral bodies to fill the space once occupied by an intervertebral disc.

Calcification (kals-see-fi-cay-shun): Body process that stimulates bone to harden.

Callus (cal-us): Granular material the body produces to mend a fracture.

Cancellous (cancel-lus): Interior compartment of bone that resembles latticework.

Cartilage (car-til-ledge): Smooth coating that covers joint surfaces.

Cartilaginous (car-t-lay-gin-us): Relating to cartilage.

Cauda Equina (caw-dah e-kwhy-nah): Lower end of the spinal cord starting near the first lumbar vertebra; structurally resembles a horse's tail.

Causalgia (cause-al-gee-ah): Severe pain that usually follows injury to a peripheral nerve.

Cerebrospinal Fluid (CSF) (sir-ee-bro-spinal fluid): Liquid cushion within the layers of the spinal cord.

Cervical Spine (sir-ve-kal spine): First seven vertebrae starting at the base of the skull abbreviated C1, C2, C3, C4, C5, C6, C7.

Chronic Pain: Constant pain described as mild to severe.

Claustrophobic (claw-stro-foe-bick): Fear of being in an enclosed space.

Clinical Symptoms: Symptoms that define a particular disorder.

Coccyx (cock-six): The tailbone; the last bone formation below the sacrum.

Collagen (call-ah-gin): Protein the body makes; helps to mend fractures.

Compression Fracture: A type of fracture that can cause a vertebra to collapse.

Compressive Neuropathy (compressive ner-row-path-ee): Pressure to nerves that may cause swelling and pain.

Computerized Axial Tomography (CT Scan or CAT Scan): A diagnostic tool that utilizes many x-ray beams to produce detailed pictures of the anatomy as 'slices'.

Congenital: A disorder that is present at birth.

Contained Disc: Also called a **Bulging Disc.** Part of the annulus of an intervertebral disc protrudes, the nucleus remains contained.

Corpectomy (core-peck-toe-me): Surgical removal of bone from the front of the neck (cervical spine).

Cortical (core-tea-cul): Outer layer of bone; structurally resembles concentric rings.

Degenerative Disc Disease (DDD): Changes associated with aging that causes discs to crack, become thin, bulge or herniate.

Dermatome (dur-ma-tome): Specific area of skin supplied by fibers from a single nerve root.

Diagnosis: Name applied to define specific disorder.

Disc (or disk): An intervertebral disc. Cushion-like shock absorber located between two vertebrae.

Discectomy (dis-eck-toe-me): Surgical removal of a portion or an entire intervertebral disc.

Discography (dis-ah-gra-fee), **Discogram:** A test that attempts to reproduce symptoms suspected to be caused by a disc.

Dorsiflex (door-see-flex): Pointing the foot or toes toward the head. The act of dorsiflexing is dorsiflexion.

Dura Mater (doo-rah matter): One of the protective membranes covering the spinal cord.

Dysesthesia (dis-ah-thee-z-ah): Abnormal or unpleasant sensations.

Electrical Stimulation or Transcutaneous Electrical Stimulation (TENS): Modality used to stimulate circulation and healing, alleviate swelling and pain.

Electrocardiogram (ECG) (electro-car-dee-oh-gram): Test used to take an electrical picture of the heart.

Electromyography (EMG) (elec-tro-mypah-gra-fee): Test used to determine if muscle function is normal.

Endoscope (en-doe-scope): Tube-like surgical instrument used to examine the inside of the body.

Endplate: Fibrocartilage structures that firmly hold each intervertebral disc between the upper and lower vertebrae.

Epidural (ep-e-do-ral): Injection of medication into the spinal canal's epidural space to alleviate symptoms.

Epidural Space (ep-e-do-ral space): Space surrounding the dura mater of the spinal cord.

Facet Joint (fah-set joint): Spinal joints.

Fascia (fay-sha): Fibrous sheets that encase muscles.

Fibrocartilage (fybro-car-til-ledge): Super strong cartilage.

Fluoroscope (floor-o-scope) or Fluoroscopy: Real time x-ray.

Foramen (foe-ray-men): Passageway where a nerve root exits the spinal canal.

Foraminal Stenosis (foe-ray-min-al sten-oh-sis): Narrowing or closing of a spinal foramen.

Foraminotomy (for-am-not-toe-me): Surgical procedure performed to increase the size the foramen or neuroforamen.

General Anesthesia (general an-es-thee-z-ah): Drugs used by an anesthesiologist during surgery that temporarily disables nerve impulses making the patient unconscious and pain free.

Hardware: Slang term for spinal instrumentation such as cages, plates, rods and screws.

Haversian Spaces (hav-er-sh-on spaces): Vascular canals in bone.

Herniated Disc (her-knee-ate-ed disc): Non-Contained Disc; the annulus breaks open allowing the nucleus pulposus to leak outside of the disc.

Hyperalgesia (hy-per-al-gee-zee-ah): Increased sensitivity to pain.

Hyperesthesia (hi-per-es-thee-zee-ah): Acute abnormal skin sensitivity.

Hyperextension (hi-per ex-ten-shun): Extension of a joint or soft tissue beyond its normal limits.

Hyperflexion (hi-per-flex-un): Flexion of a joint or soft tissue beyond its normal limits.

Hyperreflexia (hi-per-ref-flex-e-ah): Condition that causes deep tendon reflexes to become exaggerated.

Hypoalgesia (hi-poe-al-g-zee-ah): Diminished skin sensation.

Idiopathic Scoliosis (id-dee-oh-path-ick sko-lee-oh-sis): Abnormal curvature to the left or right of the spine; cause is not known.

Inflammation (in-flah-may-shun): Swelling.

Informed Consent: Full disclosure in writing about a medical procedure; requires the patient's signature.

Interspinous Ligament (in-ter-spy-nus lig-ah-ment): One of the strong fibrous connective tissues that connects spinal bone and cartilage together.

Intertransverse Ligament (in-ter-tranz-verse lig-ah-ment): One of the strong fibrous connective tissues that connects spinal vertebrae.

Intrathecal (intra-thee-cal): The fluid-containing space that surrounds the spinal cord.

Intraoperative: During surgery.

Kyphoplasty (kye-foe-plasty): Minimally invasive surgical technique using a specialized balloon and a type of medical grade cement to stabilize spinal fractures and relieve pain.

Kyphosis (kye-foe-sis): Normal or abnormal spinal curve. Abnormal forward spinal curvature is an example of abnormal kyphosis may cause a hump to form in the shoulder blade area of the upper back.

Kyphotic (kye-fah-tick): Relating to kyphosis.

Lamina (lamb-in-ah), **Laminae** (lamb-in-e, plural): Thin bony plates that protect the spinal canal.

Laminectomy (lamb-in-eck-toe-me): Surgical removal of the lamina.

Laminotomy (lamb-in-ah-toe-me): Surgical removal of a portion of the lamina.

Ligament (lig-ah-ment): Strong fibrous connective tissue that connects or joins bone, cartilage or other structures together.

Ligamentum Flavum (lig-ah-men-tum flay-vum): Yellow-colored ligament that connects the laminae to adjacent vertebrae.

Local Anesthetic (local an-es-thet-ick): Injection at or near the procedure site to block or numb nerve impulses; temporarily reduces or eliminates pain during a procedure.

Lordosis (lor-doe-sis): Normal or abnormal curvature of the spine. Swayback, an inward spinal curvature is an example of an abnormal lordosis.

Lordotic (lor-dot-ick): Relating to lordosis.

Lumbar Spine (lum-bar spine): Five or six vertebrae that follow the last thoracic vertebrae. Abbreviated L1, L2, L3, L4, L5, L6.

Lumbosacral Spine (lumbo-say-kral): Lower lumbar spine and the sacrum.

Magnetic Resonance Imaging (MRI): Diagnostic imaging tool that renders highly detailed pictures without x-ray.

Malignant (mal-eg-nant): Cancer or cancerous.

Marrow: Semi-soft center of bone where blood is produced.

Meninges (men-in-jez): Protective layers that cover the spinal cord.

Metastasize (ma-tax-ta-size): When disease (cancer) spreads to another part of the body.

Microdiscectomy (mycro-dis-eck-toe-me): Surgical removal of a portion of or an entire intervertebral disc using microscopic magnification.

Modality (mow-dal-it-tee): Passive treatment or therapy that does not require the patient's participation.

Muscle Spasm: Involuntary contraction of one or more muscles; may cause severe pain.

Musculoskeletal: Body's muscle and bone system.

Myelopathy (my-il-lop-ah-thee): Compression of or pressure on the spinal cord. May be caused by disorders such as bone spurs (osteophytes) or spinal stenosis.

Myofascial Release (my-oh-fash-e-al release): Local massage to manipulate muscle fascia.

Narcotic: Prescription drug to control pain.

Nerve Block: Injection into the area around a nerve or group of nerves to block pain impulses.

Nerve Conduction Velocity (NCV): Sensitive test to determine a nerve's ability to transit an impulse.

Nerve Root: A nerve or nerves that shoot off from the spinal cord.

Neuralgia (nu-ral-g-al): Nerve pain caused by damage or dysfunction.

Neuritis (nu-ry-tis): Nerve inflammation.

Neuroforamen (nu-row for-a-men): Small openings or passageways in the spine. Nerve roots exit the spinal canal through these structures.

Neuropathy (nu-rop-ah-thee) or Neuropathic Pain: Inflammatory process of the nerves; causes neuropathic pain.

Neurostimulation: Use of a spinal cord stimulating device to help control pain.

Neutral Spine: Denotes proper posture and use of good body mechanics to reduce unnecessary stress to the spine.

Nociceptive (no-si-sep-tive): Response to a painful stimulus; localized pain.

Non-Contained Disc: See Herniated Disc.

Nucleus Pulposus (new-klee-us pul-poe-sis): Gel-like center of an intervertebral disc.

Nuclide (noo-clid): Radioactive tracer.

Odontoid Process (oh-don-toyed process): Tooth-like projection, part of the axis.

Opiate, Opioid (oh-pe-ate, oh-pe-oid): Pain drug chemically related to opium.

Ossification (os-efik-kay-shun): The development of bone.

Osteoarthritis (OA). (os-t-o-arth-rye-tis): A degenerative form of arthritis.

Osteoblast (os-t-o-blast): A bone-forming cell.

Osteoclast (os-t-o-kast): A cell that absorbs and removes bone.

Osteocyte (os-t-o-site): A mature bone-forming cell (osteoblast).

Osteophyte (os-t-o-fight): Bony overgrowth, bone spur; abnormal outward growth of bone.

Osteoporosis (os-t-o-pour-o-sis): Metabolic disease that robs bones of their strength and density; may increase the risk for fracture.

Outpatient Surgery: Same day surgery.

Palpation (pal-pay-shun): The method of examining the body using touch.

Paralysis (pa-ral-eh-sis): Loss of function; inability to move and/or feel.

Paresthesia (par-s-thee-z-ah): Abnormal sensations such as tingling or pins and needles.

Pars Articularis (parz are-tick-you-lar-es): Part of the posterior vertebra including the facet joints that attach to the vertebral body.

Patient-Controlled Analgesia (PCA): Patient operated pump to self-dose pain medication after surgery.

Pedicle: The bony process that projects backward from the vertebra connecting the lamina on either side.

Percutaneous Surgery (per-cue-tay-nee-us surgery): Surgery performed through small keyhole-sized incisions in the skin.

Peripheral Neuropathy (pe-rif-er-al nu-rop-ah-thee): Disease affecting the nerves that branch into the extremities (e.g. arms, legs).

Physical Therapy: Non-surgical, conservative treatments used before or after surgery to help the patient build strength, increase range of motion and flexibility.

Pia Mater (pee-ah-matter): One of the membranes (meninges) that protect the spinal cord.

Posterior (pose-tear-e-or): Rear, behind.

Posterior Longitudinal Ligament: Spinal ligament that runs vertically behind the vertebrae to support and reinforce the intervertebral discs.

Pseudoarthrosis (sue-do-arth-roe-sis): Failed fusion.

Radiate (ray-dee-ate): Pain or sensation that travels away from the point of origin.

Radiculopathy (rah-dick-u-lop-ah-thee): Pain caused by injury to a nerve root.

Radiograph: Abbreviated x-ray.

Recovery Room: Area supervised by medical personnel where a patient is taken immediately after surgery.

Referred Pain: Pain felt in a part of the body separate from the origin of the pain.

Rheumatoid Arthritis (RA) (room-ah-toyed arth-rye-tis): Progressive form of arthritis that may be painfully destructive.

Rootlet (root-let): A nerve root that shoots off from the spinal cord.

Ruptured Disc: See Herniated Disc.

Sacral (say-kral): Relating to the sacrum.

Sacroiliac (say-kro-ill-e-ak): Relating to the sacrum, such as the sacroiliac joint (a joint in the sacrum).

Sacrum (say-krum): Triangular-shaped bone mass located below the last lumbar vertebra.

Sciatica (sy-attic-ka): A symptom indicating a compressive or inflammatory process involving the sciatic nerve; typically causes buttock and leg pain.

Scoliosis (sko-lee-oh-sis): Abnormal curvature of the spine; causes the spine to curve in the shape of an S or C.

Slipped Disc: An erroneous term used to mean bulging or herniated disc.

Soft Tissue Injury: Injury to tendons, ligaments, muscles (non-bone structures).

Spinal Fusion and Spinal Instrumentation: Surgical procedures using bone graft and cages, plates, rods or screws to stabilize the spine.

Spinal Meningitis (spinal men-in-ji-tis): Serious infection that causes inflammation of the membranes in the brain and spinal cord.

Spinal Stenosis (spinal sten-oh-sis): Narrowing or closing of the spinal canal or neuroforamen causing nerve root compression, pain and neurologic symptoms.

Spinal Tumor: Rare, abnormal growth; benign or malignant (cancerous). Tumors may be classified as Primary or Secondary.

Spondylolisthesis (spon-de-low-lis-thee-sis): A structural disorder that occurs when one vertebra slips over the adjacent vertebra below. May be classified as Developmental or Acquired.

Spondylosis (spon-dee-low-sis): Degenerative spinal arthritis that affects the intervertebral disc and facet joints.

Sprain or Strain: Hyperextension or hyperflexion; occurs when a joint or soft tissue is stretched beyond its normal limits.

Supraspinous Ligament (sue-pra-spine-us lig-ah-ment): See ligament.

Synovial Fluid (si-n-vee-al fluid): A body fluid that lubricates and nourishes joints and cartilage.

Tailbone: Last bone formation below the sacrum; the coccyx.

Tendon (ten-dun): Sturdy fibrous band of tissue that attaches muscle to bone.

Thoracic Spine (thor-as-ick spine): The 12 vertebrae following the last cervical vertebra abbreviated T1 through T12.

Transforaminal (trans- foe-ray-men-al): Surgical approach from the side of the body to the spine.

Trigger Point Injection: Injection of pain-relieving or numbing medication at the site of pain.

Ultrasound: A passive modality used to relax muscles, increase circulation and promote healing.

Urinalysis (yu-ri-nal-is-sis): Urine test.

Vertebra (ver-ta-bra). Singular: Spinal bone.

Vertebrae (ver-ta-bray): Plural form of vertebra.

Vertebral (ver-tee-brawl): Relating to a vertebra or vertebrae.

Vertebroplasty (ver-tee-bro-plasty): Minimally invasive surgical technique using a type of medical grade cement to stabilize spinal fractures and reduce pain.

Wedge Fracture: Similar to a compression fracture, the fractured vertebra resembles a wedge.

Whiplash: Intensive neck sprain/strain injury to the soft neck tissue.

X-Ray: Radiograph; common diagnostic imaging tool that uses radiation.

Zygapophyseal Joint (zye-gap-o-fiz-e-all joints): Facet joint.

Product Contributors

Advanced Neuromodulation Systems, Inc.
6901 Preston Road
Plano, TX 75024 USA
Telephone: 972-309-8000
Fax: 972-309-8150
Website: *www.ans-medical.com*

Aesculap, Inc.
3773 Corporate Parkway
Center Valley, PA 18034 USA
Telephone: 800-282-9000
Website: *www.aesculap-usa.com*

ArthroCare Spine
680 Vaqueros Avenue
Sunnyvale, CA 94085-35523 USA
Telephone: 408-736-0224
Fax: 408-736-0226
Website: *www.arthrocare.com*

Aspen Medical Products
6481 Oak Canyon
Irvine, CA 92618 USA
Telephone: 949-681-0200 or 800-295-2776
Fax: 800-848-7455
Website: *www.aspenmp.com*

Blackstone Medical, Inc.
90 Brookdale Drive
Springfield, MA 01104 USA
Telephone: 888-298-5700

Fax: 800-861-9363
Website: *www.blackstonemedical.com*

Chattanooga Group
A Division of Encore Medical Corporation
9800 Metric Boulevard
Austin, TX 78758 USA
Telephone: 800-592-7329
Website: *www.chattgroup.com*

DePuy Spine, Inc.
A Johnson & Johnson Company
325 Paramount Drive
Raynham, MD 02767 USA
Telephone: 800-227-6633
Website: *www.depuyspine.com*

EBI
100 Interpace Parkway
Parsippany, NJ 07054 USA
Telephone: 800-526-2579
Website: *www.ebimedical.com*

Encore Medical Corporation
9800 Metric Boulevard
Austin, TX 78758 USA
Telephone: 512-832-9500
Website: *www.encoremed.com*

GE Healthcare
Chalfont St. Giles
Buckinghamshire, UK
Website: *www.gehealthcare.com*

IsoTis OrthoBiologics, Inc.
2 Goodyear
Irvine, CA 92618 USA
Customer Service: 949-595-8710 or 800-550-7115
Fax: 949-595-8711 or 800-471-3248
Website: *www.isotis.com*
Rue de Sébeillon 1-3
1004 Lausanne
Switzerland
Customer Service: +41 21 620 6020
Fax: +41 21 620 6021

Kyphon Inc.
1221 Crossman Avenue
Sunnyvale, CA 94089 USA
Website: *www.kyphon.com*

Medtronic Sofamor Danek
1800 Pyramid Place
Memphis, TN 38132 USA
Website: *www.sofamordanek.com*

Neurometrics
205 JFK Drive
Atlantis, FL 33462 USA
Telephone: 561-432-5888 or 877-584-5100
Fax: 561-432-5599
Email: *iom@neurometrics.info*

Orthofix, Inc.
1720 Bray Central Drive
McKinney, TX 75069 USA
Telephone: 469-742-2500
Website: *www.orthofix.com*

OrthoVita, Inc.
45 Great Valley Parkway
Malvern, PA 19355 USA
Telephone: 610-640-1775
Website: *www.orthovita.com*

Relax The Back
Over 100 Stores Nationwide
Telephone: 888-Relax59
Website: *www.relaxtheback.com*

Spinal Concepts
An Abbott Laboratories Company
5301 Riata Park Court
Building F
Austin, TX 78727 USA
Telephone: 512-918-2700
Website: *www.spinalconcepts.com*

Stryker Spine
2 Pearl Court
Allendale, NJ 07401 USA
Telephone: 877-946-9678
Fax: 201-831-6287
Website: *www.strykerspine.com*

Synthes Spine
P.O. Box 1766
1690 Russell Road
Paoli, PA 19301 USA
Telephone: 610 647 9700
Fax: 800 345 1272
Website: *www.synthes.com*

Tempur-Pedic International Inc.
1713 Jaggie Fox Way
Lexington, KY 40511 USA
Telephone: 800-878-8889
Website: *www.tempurpedic.com*

Zimmer Spine, Inc.
7375 Bush Lake Road
Minneapolis, MN 55439-2027 USA
Telephone: 952-832-5600 or 800-655-2614
Fax: 952-832-5620
Website: *www.zimmerspine.com*

Index

Index

Index

H

Hardware. *See* instrumentation
Haversian space, 19–20
Heat therapy, 224–25, 244
Herniated disc (ruptured disc), 2, 41–42,
    46, 47, 53, 77, 78, 96, 103, 106,
    162, 166–67, 175, 176, 234
Hydrotherapy, 225, 244
Hyperextension, 30–31
Hyperflexion, 30–31
Hyperreflexia, 99

I-J

Ice therapy, 59, 225, 244
Idiopathic scoliosis, 38
Image-guided surgery, 153
Infection, 2, 7, 10, 33, 69, 71, 91, 116
Informed consent, 73
INFUSE® Bone Graft, 144–46,
Injection, 32, 37, 42, 46, 53, 63, 65, 71,
    76, 92, 106, 110–11, 162, 176, 242,
    243–44, 248, 249–50
Instrumentation, 79–80, 82, 83–87,
    123–31, 152, 156, 172, 214–15,
Intelect® Portable Electrotherapy, 65–66
Interbody cage. *See* cage
Intersegmental system, 26
Interspinous ligament, 27
Intertransverse ligament, 27
Intervertebral disc, 10, 11–12, 20, 22–23,
    26, 32, 40–42, 44, 46, 77, 83, 94,
    95, 98, 105, 106, 109–10, 144, 175,
    187, 188, 191
Intradiscal electrothermoplasty (IDET),
    245
Intrasegmental system, 26
Intrathecal, 242, 246

K

Kyphoplasty, 36, 178–82
Kyphosis, kyphotic, 21, 38–39, 86, 128

L

Laboratory tests, 10
Laminectomy, 54, 78, 162, 173

Laminotomy, 78–79, 107
Leg pain, 37, 71, 141, 142, 150, 167, 175,
    234, 247, 262–63
Ligament, 26–27, 29–30, 40, 45, 67, 166
Ligamentum flavum, 26, 27
Lordosis, lordotic, 21, 39, 145, 223
LT-CAGE® Lumbar Tapered Fusion
    Device, 144–46
Lumbar, 20, 21, 22, 23, 31, 33, 36, 37,
    45–46, 47, 50, 69, 80, 127–30, 133,
    136, 138–47, 150, 158, 159,
    160–61, 172, 191–93, 195, 213,
    214, 215, 217, 234, 243

M

Magnetic resonance imaging (MRI), 10,
    11–13, 15–17, 33, 48, 49, 52, 100
MAVERICK™ Total Disc Replacement,
    195–96
Medial branch block, 250
Medication, drugs, 30, 32, 33, 36, 37, 42,
    44, 53, 57, 62–63, 67, 71, 75, 76,
    92, 101, 108–9, 111, 162, 167–68,
    230, 243–44, 246, 248–56
MEH4™ Titanium Mesh Vertebral Body
    Replacement, 136–37
Meninges, 23, 24, 25
Meningitis, spinal meningitis, 33, 98
Metastatic tumor, 67
METRx™ MicroDiscectomy System,
    169–71
Microdiscectomy, 77, 169–71
MicroEndoscopic Discectomy (MED),
    162–65
Minimally invasive, 73, 77–79, 149–86
Muscle, 19, 26–33, 57, 58, 62, 65, 68, 97,
    151, 156, 164, 168, 222, 224, 225,
    226, 243–44
Muscle spasm, 30, 33, 37, 43, 47, 57, 59,
    65, 167–68, 224, 225
Musculoskeletal, 19
Myelopathy, 98
Myofascial release, 225

Index

Index

Rheumatoid arthritis (RA), 44, 69, 91, 97–98, 251, 252, 253

Romberg test, 4

S

Sacral, sacrum, 20, 21, 22, 44, 127, 130, 161, 211

Sciatic nerve, 31–32

Sciatica, 31–32, 49, 160, 175, 245

Scoliosis, 2, 37–38, 77, 79, 83, 86, 87, 127, 128, 212, 247

Secondary tumor, 49

Selective nerve root block, 250

Signa OpenSpeed 0.7T: Magnetic Resonance Imaging, 15–16

Skeleton, 19

Slipped disc, 40

Smoking, 48, 72

Soft tissue disorders, 11, 14, 29–33, 43, 52, 59, 253

SpF® Spinal Fusion Stimulator, 214–16

Spinal canal, 25, 31, 41, 44–45, 63, 78, 100, 182, 263, 264

Spinal column, 20, 21, 22, 53, 64, 133

Spinal cord, 11, 23, 24–26, 27, 28, 33, 34, 35, 40, 45, 46, 51, 53, 64, 93, 96, 98, 100–103, 108, 208, 242, 244, 246–47, 254

Spinal cord stimulator, 65, 242, 256–62

Spinal disorders, 2, 7, 29–51, 71, 127, 146, 207–9, 212

Spinal pump, 246, 247

Spinal stenosis, 44–46, 47, 50–55, 78, 113, 123, 141, 142, 182, 234, 241, 243, 247

Spinal-Stim® Lite, 216–18

Spine specialist, 1–5, 7, 14, 37, 49–50, 54, 72, 84, 176, 212, 251

Spondylolisthesis, 36–37, 39, 45, 47, 79, 85, 127, 128, 141–42, 146, 150, 172, 182, 212, 234

Spondylosis, 92, 96–97, 99, 107–8

Sprain, strain, 7, 29, 30, 65, 241, 251

Stabilizer™ Pressure Biofeedback, 231–32

Supine, 4

Supraspinous ligament, 27

Surgery, 38, 44, 46, 54, 65, 71–89, 101–3, 106–7, 111–58, 162–67, 169–209, 214–16

Surgical conference, 73

Sympathetic nerve block, 244

T

Tailbone, coccyx, 20, 21, 263, 264

Tempur-Pedic Swedish Sleep Systems®, 235–37

Tendon, 26, 27, 29–30, 252

TheraTherm® Digital Moist Heating Pad, 59–61

Thoracic, 20, 21, 22, 23, 123–27, 130, 133, 136, 211, 212, 213, 252

Trabecular Metal™ Material, 203–4

Traction, 57–59, 67–70, 109

Transcutaneous electrical stimulation (TENS). *See* electrical stimulation

Transforaminal lumbar interbody fusion (TLIF), 180

Trigger point injection, 242, 243–44

Tumor, 2, 7, 10, 35, 48–49, 52, 53, 69, 71, 86, 98, 123, 128, 130, 133

U

Ultrasound, 61, 65, 225, 226

V

Vascular system, 27–28

Vertebra, vertebrae, vertebral, 20, 21, 22, 23, 25, 28, 31, 33, 36, 86, 92–93, 95, 102, 142, 144, 161, 172, 174, 179, 180, 182

Vertebral arches, 24

Vertebral column, 20, 86, 184

Vertebroplasty, 36, 179

VITOSS™ Synthetic Cancellous Bone, 205–6

VueCath® System: Spinal Endoscopic Tool, 262–64

W

Whiplash, 30–31, 58, 97, 212, 251

Index

X-Y

X-Ray, 7, 9, 10, 11–12, 13–14, 30, 34, 38, 43, 44, 47, 52, 53, 63, 74, 79, 140, 152, 163, 179, 196

Xia® Spinal System, 130–31

Z

Zero-Gravity Perfect Chair, 238–39

Zygapophyseal joint, 23